Instructor's Manual for Administering Medications

Pharmacology for Health Careers

Fifth Edition

Donna F. Gauwitz, R.N., M.S.
Senior Teaching Specialist
University of Minnesota
Minneapolis, Minnesota

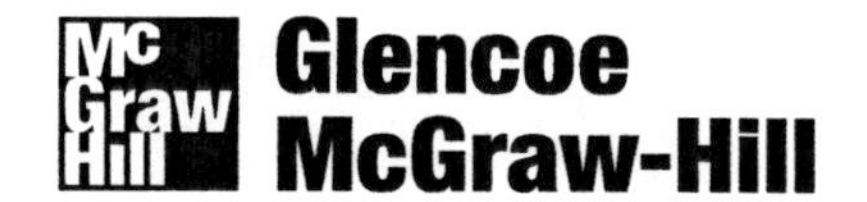

New York, New York
Columbus, Ohio
Woodland Hills, California
Peoria, Illinois

Send all inquiries to:
Glencoe/McGraw-Hill
936 Eastwind Drive
Westerville, OH 43081

ISBN-13: 978-0-07-297453-9
ISBN-10: 0-07-297453-2

Part of

ISBN-13: 978-0-07-297514-7
ISBN-10: 0-07-297514-8

4 5 6 7 8 9 10 066 09 08 07 06

Contents

Preface

The Instructor's Manual provides you with materials to help organize classroom lessons and interactions. It includes the following:

- A list of chapter objectives
- A chapter outline
- Teaching strategies
- Critical thinking activities
- Answers to the chapter review
- Answers to the chapter tests
- Chapter tests

New to this edition are correlation charts. The material presented in the student textbook are correlated with the following:

- AAMA Role Delineation Study Areas of Competence
- The AMT Registered Medical Assistant (RMA) Certification Exam Topics
- SCANS (Secretary's Commission on Achieving Necessary Skills)
- The National Health Care Skill Standards

Also new to this edition is the inclusion of the Instructor's Presentation Software and test bank. The presentation software contains PowerPoint transparencies to help you illustrate and review key points from each chapter of the student textbook. Included on the transparencies are a review of key terms, questions to prompt classroom discussion, and critical thinking activities. The test bank will allow you to create your own tests to measure students' knowledge of chapter concepts. It contains numerous test layout and printing options and the capability to edit and add questions.

Together, the Instructor's Manual and the student textbook form a complete teaching and learning package. *Administering Medications: Pharmacology for Health Careers* will prepare the student to enter the health care field with the knowledge and skills necessary to become a useful resource to patients and a valued asset to employers.

Instructor's Presentation and Student Assessment Software

ExamView TEST GENERATOR INTRODUCTION

These instructions accompany a test generator program called *ExamView*—an application that enables you to quickly and easily create tests, enter your own questions, and customize the appearance of the tests you create. The *ExamView* test generator program offers many unique features. Using the QuickTest wizard, for example, you are guided step-by-step through the process of building a test. Numerous options are included that allow you to customize the content and appearance of the tests you create.

As you work with the *ExamView* test generator, you may use the following features:

- **an interview mode or "wizard" to guide you through the steps to create a test in less than five minutes**
- **five methods to select test questions**
  - from a list
  - random selection
  - by criteria (difficulty code or objective–if available)
  - while viewing questions
  - all questions
- **the capability to edit questions or to add an unlimited number of questions**
- **a sophisticated word processor**
  - streamlined question entry
  - toolbar
  - cut, copy, paste, undo
  - tabs (center, left, right, decimal, leaders)
  - fonts and text styles (bold, underline, color, etc.)
  - support for symbols and foreign characters
  - tables
  - borders and shading
  - paragraph formatting (justification, spacing, hanging indent, etc.)
  - pictures or other graphics within a question, answer, or narrative
  - find/replace commands
- **numerous test layout and printing options**
  - scramble the choices in multiple choice questions
  - organize matching questions in a one- or two-column format
  - print multiple versions of the same test with corresponding answer keys
  - print an answer key strip for easier test grading
  - change the order of questions
  - print a test with or without space for students to record their answers
  - specify the layout of a test to conserve paper
  - print a comprehensive answer sheet
- **the ability to link groups of questions to common narratives**
- **password protection**
- **extensive help system**

ExamView INSTALLATION AND START-UP INSTRUCTIONS

The *ExamView* test generator software is provided on one or more floppy disks or on a CD-ROM depending on the question bank. The disks include the program and all of the questions for the corresponding textbook. Before you can use the test generator software, you must install it on your hard drive or network. The system requirements, installation instructions, and startup procedures are provided below.

SYSTEM REQUIREMENTS

To use the *ExamView* test generator, your computer must meet or exceed these minimum hardware requirements:

- 486, 50 MHz computer
- Windows 3.1, Windows 95, Windows 98, or Windows NT
- color monitor (VGA-compatible)
- high-density floppy disk drive
- hard drive with at least 5 MB space available
- 8 MB available memory *(16 MB memory recommended)*
- mouse
- printer

INSTALLATION INSTRUCTIONS

Follow these steps to install the *ExamView* test generator software on a hard drive or network. The setup program will automatically install everything you need to use the *ExamView* test generator software.

Step 1
Turn on your computer.

Step 2
Insert the *ExamView* installation disk into Drive A. If the program is provided on a CD-ROM, insert the disc into your CD-ROM drive.

Step 3
Windows 3.1: While in the Program Manager, choose *Run* from the **File** menu.
Windows 95/98: Click the **Start** button on the *Taskbar* and choose the *Run* option.

Step 4
If you are installing the software from floppy disks, type **a:\setup** and press **Enter** to run the installation program. If the *ExamView* software is provided on a CD-ROM, use the drive letter that corresponds to the CD-ROM drive on your computer (e.g., **e:\setup** or **e:\examview\setup**).

Note: The installation program is configured to copy the software to *c:\examview* on your hard drive. You can, however, change this location. For example, you can select a location on your network server.

Step 5
Follow the prompts on the screen to complete the installation process. If the software and question banks are provided on more than one disk, you will be prompted to insert the appropriate disk when it is needed.

Step 6
Remove the installation disk from the disk drive when you finish.

GETTING STARTED

After you complete the installation process, follow these instructions to start the *ExamView* software. This section also explains the options used to create a test and edit a question bank.

Start-Up Instructions

Step 1
Turn on the computer.

Step 2

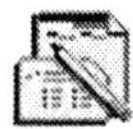

Windows 3.1: Locate the *ExamView* program icon. Double-click the program icon to start the test generator software.
Windows 95/98: Click the **Start** button on the *Taskbar.* Highlight the **Programs** menu and locate the *ExamView* folder. Select the *ExamView* option to start the software.

Step 3
The first time you run the software you will be prompted to enter your name, school/institution name, and city/state. You are now ready to begin using the *ExamView* software.

Step 4
Each time you start *ExamView,* the **Startup** menu appears. As shown in Figure 1, choose one of the following options:

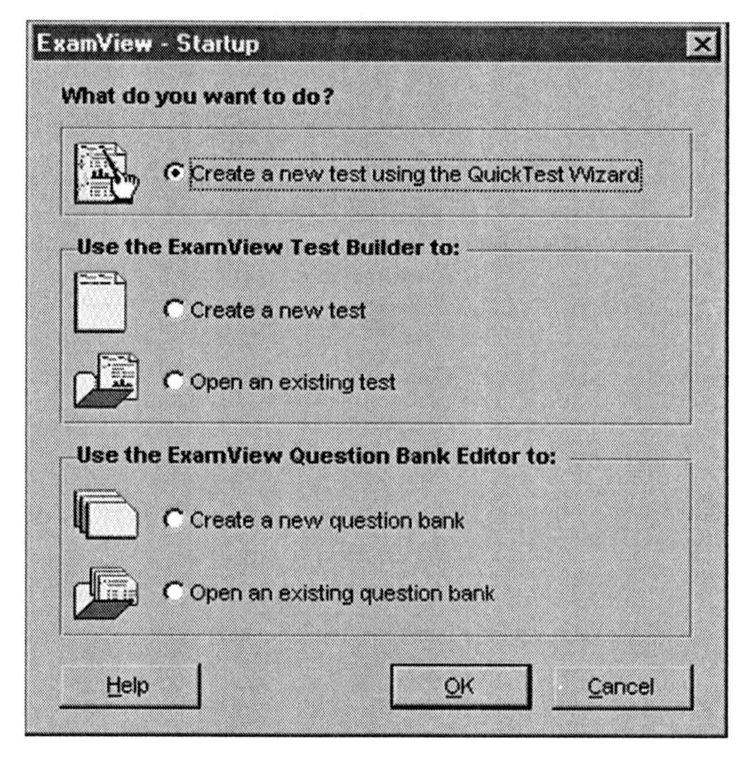

Figure 1 – ExamView Startup Menu

Step 5
Use *ExamView* to create a test or edit questions in a question bank.

The *ExamView* program is divided into two components: Test Builder and Question Bank Editor. The **Test Builder** includes options to create, edit, print, and save tests. The **Question Bank Editor** lets you create or edit existing question banks. Both the Test Builder and the Question Bank Editor have unique menus and options to work with tests and question banks.

As you work with *ExamView,* you can easily switch between these components using the *Switch to...* option in the **File** menu. Be sure to save your work before you switch between components.

Important: Whenever you need assistance using *ExamView,* access the extensive help system. Click the **Help** button or choose an option from the **Help** menu to access step-by-step instructions and detailed descriptions of the features of *ExamView.* If you experience any difficulties while you are working with the software, you may want to review the troubleshooting tips in the user-friendly help system.

Test Builder

The Test Builder will empower you to create tests using the QuickTest Wizard or you can create a new test on your own.

- *If you want ExamView to choose questions randomly from one or more question banks,* choose the QuickTest Wizard option to create a new test. Then, follow the step-by-step instructions to (1) enter a test title, (2) choose the question bank from which to select questions, and (3) identify how many questions you want on the test. The QuickTest Wizard will automatically create a new test and use the Test Builder to display the test on screen. You can print the test as is, remove questions, add new questions, or edit any questions.
- *If you want to create a new test on your own,* choose the option to create a new test. Then identify a question bank from which to choose questions by using the *Question Bank* option in the **Select** menu. You may then add questions to the test by using one or more of the following question selection options: *Randomly, From a List, While Viewing, By Criteria,* or *All Questions.*

After you create a test, you can customize the appearance of the test by changing the order of the questions, editing test instructions, specifying the font and style for selected test elements, and choosing whether to leave space for students to write their answers directly on the test. The customizing changes you make to the questions will not change the original question bank; your changes are made only to the copy of the questions on the test you just created.

When you have finalized the content and appearance of your test, you can print it and/or save it. To print a test, you may choose how many copies of the test you want, whether you want all the copies to be the same, and whether you want to scramble the questions and the multiple choice options. If you scramble the questions, *ExamView* will print a custom answer sheet for each variation of the test.

Question Bank Editor

The Question Bank Editor will empower you to edit questions in an existing publisher-supplied question bank or to create new question banks. Always use the Question Bank Editor if you want to change a question permanently in an existing question bank.

You may edit questions in a question bank or add new questions by using the built-in word processor. The word processor includes many features commonly found in commercially available word processing applications. These features include the following: fonts, styles, tables, paragraph formatting, ruler controls, tabs, indents, and justification.

A question bank may include up to 250 questions in a variety of formats including multiple choice, true/false, modified true/false, completion, yes/no, matching, problem, essay, short answer, case, and numeric response. You can assign a difficulty code, a page reference, and two objectives to each question.

SOFTWARE SUPPORT

McGraw-Hill provides toll-free telephone assistance for instructors who experience difficulty while using *ExamView.* Before calling for assistance, please check the following:

- Is your computer working properly? Try some other software, which you know is working, on the same computer.
- Are you certain the software is working properly? Try the software on another computer.
- Can you repeat the problem? Does the problem occur at the same point each time?

In order for the Support Center to help you as quickly as possible, before calling for assistance have the following at hand:

- exact title and ISBN number from the disk label or package.
- brand, model, and configuration of the computer you are using.
- system version (Windows 3.1, Windows 95, or Windows 98) installed on your computer.
- the exact wording of any error message.

The McGraw-Hill Support Center toll-free number is **800-437-3715.** The Support Center is available from 8:00 A.M. to 6:00 P.M. Eastern Standard Time. You can also send an E-mail to the following address **epgtech@mcgraw-hill.com** to contact the Support Center.

INSTRUCTOR PRESENTATION SOFTWARE

The Instructor Presentation Software CD-ROM, located on the inside back cover of this Instructor's Manual, contains additional review material, questions, and case studies as PowerPoint slides and the PowerPoint Viewer. You will find one presentation per chapter. The PowerPoint Viewer is a program used to run slide shows on computers that do not have the full PowerPoint program installed.

If you have PowerPoint 97 (or higher) it is not necessary to install the PowerPoint Viewer in order to view the slides. Also, PowerPoint 97 allows you to modify the presentations if you desire.

PowerPoint Viewer Installation Instructions

To install the PowerPoint Viewer use the instructions that follow. Please note that Windows 95 (or higher) is required to run the PowerPoint Viewer. Also, a display setting of 640 × 480, or 800 × 600 is strongly recommended.

1. Insert the disc into the CD-ROM drive.
2. Click the START menu button and choose the RUN option.
3. Type E:\PPVIEW97 and press ENTER. (Note: Use the appropriate drive letter that corresponds with your CD-ROM drive.)
4. Follow the instructions on the screen to complete the installation process. (Note: You must install the PowerPoint Viewer onto your hard drive.)

Start-Up Instructions

Use the following steps to start the PowerPoint Viewer program and open a presentation file:

1. Click the START menu button and choose the PROGRAMS option.
2. Select MICROSOFT POWERPOINT VIEWER 97 to start the program.
3. Click the LOOK IN: pop-up menu and select your CD-ROM drive.
4. Double-click on the folder name CHAPTERS to open the folder that contains the presentations for each chapter.
5. Choose a chapter (for example, click CHAP1.PPT, then click OPEN).
6. While viewing a case presentation, press the SPACE BAR to move to the next slide or click the left mouse button. Use the PgUp key to go to the previous slide.
7. To exit the presentation, press the ESC (Escape) key.

AAMA Role Delineation Study Areas of Competence (1997) Correlation Chart

Areas of Competence	Student Edition
I. Administrative	
A. Administrative Procedures	
1. Perform basic clerical functions.	
2. Schedule, coordinate, and monitor appointments.	
3. Schedule inpatient/outpatient admissions and procedures.	
4. Understand and apply third-party guidelines.	
5. Obtain reimbursement through accurate claims submission.	
6. Monitor third-party reimbursement.	
7. Perform medical transcription.	
8. Understand and adhere to managed care policies and procedures.	
* Negotiate managed care contracts.	
B. Practice Finances	
1. Perform procedural and diagnostic coding.	
2. Apply bookkeeping principles.	
3. Document and maintain accounting and banking records.	
4. Manage accounts receivable.	
5. Manage accounts payable.	
6. Process payroll.	
* Develop and maintain fee schedules.	
* Manage personnel benefits and maintain records.	
II. Clinical	
A. Fundamental Principles	
1. Apply principles of aseptic technique and infection control.	
2. Comply with quality assurance practices.	
3. Screen and follow up patient test results.	
B. Diagnostic Orders	
1. Collect and process specimens.	
2. Perform diagnostic tests.	
C. Patient Care	
1. Adhere to established triage procedures.	
2. Obtain patient history and vital signs.	
3. Prepare and maintain examination and treatment areas.	
4. Prepare patient for examinations, procedures, and treatments.	4–20
5. Assist with examinations, procedures, and treatments.	4–20
6. Prepare and administer medications and immunizations.	4–20

* Advanced skill

AAMA Role Delineation Study Areas of Competence (1997) Correlation Chart (cont.)

Areas of Competence	Student Edition
7. Maintain medication and immunization records.	4–20
8. Recognize and respond to emergencies.	
9. Coordinate patient care information with other health care providers.	4
III. General (Transdisciplinary)	
A. Professionalism	
1. Project a professional manner and image.	
2. Adhere to ethical principles.	1, 2, 4
3. Demonstrate initiative and responsibility.	
4. Work as a team member.	1, 4
5. Manage time effectively.	
6. Prioritize and perform multiple tasks.	
7. Adapt to change.	
8. Promote the CMA credential.	
9. Enhance skills through continuing education.	
B. Communication Skills	
1. Treat all patients with compassion and empathy.	5–20
2. Recognize and respect cultural diversity.	5–20
3. Adapt communications to individual's ability to understand.	5–20
4. Use professional telephone technique.	
5. Use effective and correct verbal and written communications.	4–20
6. Recognize and respond to verbal and nonverbal communications.	5–20
7. Use medical terminology appropriately.	1–20
8. Receive, organize, prioritize, and transmit information.	1–20
9. Serve as a liaison.	
10. Promote the practice through positive public relations.	
C. Legal Concepts	
1. Maintain confidentiality.	1
2. Practice within the scope of education, training, and personal capabilities.	1
3. Prepare and maintain medical records.	1, 4
4. Document accurately.	1, 4
5. Use appropriate guidelines when releasing information.	1, 4
6. Follow employer's established policies dealing with the health care contract.	
7. Follow federal, state, and local legal guidelines.	1, 4
8. Maintain awareness of federal and state health care legislation and regulations.	1, 4

AAMA Role Delineation Study Areas of Competence (1997) Correlation Chart (cont.)

Areas of Competence	Student Edition
9. Maintain and dispose of regulated substances in compliance with government guidelines.	1, 4
10. Comply with established risk management and safety procedures.	1, 4
11. Recognize professional credentialing criteria.	
12. Participate in the development and maintenance of personnel, policy, and procedure manuals.	
* Develop and maintain personnel, policy, and procedure manuals.	
D. Instruction	
1. Instruct individuals according to their needs.	5–20
2. Explain office policies and procedures.	
3. Teach methods of health promotion and disease prevention.	5–20
4. Locate community resources and disseminate information.	
* Develop educational materials.	
* Conduct continuing education activities.	
E. Operational Functions	
1. Maintain supply inventory.	
2. Evaluate and recommend equipment and supplies.	
3. Apply computer techniques to support office operations.	
* Negotiate leases and prices for equipment and supply contracts.	

* Advanced skill

AMT Registered Medical Assistant (RMA) Certification Exam Topics Correlation Chart

Exam Topics	Student Edition
I. General Medical Assisting Knowledge	
A. Anatomy & Physiology	
1. Body systems—Know the structure and function of the: Skeletal system, Muscular system, Endocrine system, Urinary system, Reproductive system, Gastrointestinal system, Nervous system, Respiratory system, Cardiovascular system, Integumentary system, Special senses system	1, 6–19
2. Disorders of the body—Identify various diseases, conditions, and syndromes.	6–20
B. Medical Terminology	
1. Word parts—Identify word parts—root, prefixes, and suffixes.	
2. Definitions—Define medical terms.	1–20
3. Common abbreviations and symbols—Know medical abbreviations and symbols.	1, 2, 3, 4
4. Spelling—Spell medical terms correctly.	1–20
C. Medical Law	
1. Medical law—Identify the various types of consent, and how and when to obtain each; know disclosure laws (i.e., what information must be reported to proper agency); what constitutes confidential information; what information may be disclosed under certain circumstances; recognize legal responsibilities of the medical assistant; know the various medically related laws (i.e., Good Samaritan, Anatomical Gift Act, drug storage and record maintenance, Drug Enforcement Agency Regulations).	1, 2, 4
2. Licensure, certification, and registration—Know credentialing requirements of medical professionals.	
D. Medical Ethics	
1. Principles of medical ethics—Know the principles of medical ethics established by the American Medical Association; define terminology associated with medical ethics.	1, 2, 4
2. Ethical conduct—Identify the ethical response for the various situations in a medical facility; recognize unethical practices.	1, 2, 4
E. Human Relations	
1. Patient relations—Identify emotional reactions of various age groups; respond appropriately to emotional needs of patients.	6–20
2. Other interpersonal relations—Employ appropriate interpersonal skills in the workplace.	6–20

AMT Registered Medical Assistant (RMA) Certification Exam Topics Correlation Chart (cont.)

Exam Topics	Student Edition
F. Patient Education	
1. Patient instruction—Employ various methods to instruct patients (i.e., echo method, verbal, and written instructions); instruct patients, as directed, in areas of nutrition, diet, medications, body mechanics, and treatment procedures; document patient instruction properly.	6–20
2. Patient resource materials—Maintain patient resource materials.	
II. Administrative Medical Assisting	
A. Insurance	
1. Terminology—Assist patients with insurance inquiries; know terminology associated with health and accident insurance in the medical office.	
2. Plans—Know the major types of medical insurance programs encountered in the medical office, including government-sponsored, group, individual, and workers' compensation programs.	
3. Claim forms—Complete and file forms for insurance claims; evaluate claims rejection; complete "first" reports.	
4. Coding—Know coding systems used in insurance processing; code diagnoses and procedures.	
5. Financial aspects of medical insurance—Know billing requirements for insurance programs; process insurance payments; track unpaid claims.	
B. Financial Bookkeeping	
1. Terminology—Know terminology associated with financial bookkeeping in the medical office.	
2. Patient billing—Maintain and explain physician's fee schedules; collect and post payments; manage patient ledgers; make financial arrangements with patients; prepare and mail itemized statements; know methods of billing; cycle billing procedures.	
3. Collections—Identify delinquent accounts; take appropriate steps for collection; perform skip tracing; perform telephone collection procedures; know collection as related to bankruptcy and small claims cases.	
4. Fundamental medical office accounting procedures—Employ appropriate accounting procedures (e.g., pegboard); employ daily balancing procedures; prepare monthly trial balance; know accounts payable/receivable.	
5. Banking—Manage petty cash; prepare and make bank deposits; reconcile bank statements; use and process checks appropriately (including NSF and endorsement requirements); maintain checking account; process payables (office bills).	

AMT Registered Medical Assistant (RMA) Certification Exam Topics Correlation Chart (cont.)

Exam Topics	Student Edition
6. Employee payroll—Prepare employee payroll; maintain payroll tax deduction records; prepare employee tax forms; prepare payroll tax deduction reports; know terminology pertaining to payroll and taxes.	
7. Financial mathematics—Perform calculations related to patient and practice accounts.	
C. Medical Secretarial-Receptionist	
1. Terminology—Know terminology associated with medical secretarial and receptionist duties.	
2. Reception—Receive and greet patients and visitors under nonemergency conditions; screen visitors and sales persons requesting to see physician; obtain patient information; call/assist patients into examination room.	
3. Scheduling—Employ appointment scheduling system (maintain appointment book, type daily schedule, review schedule with physician); prepare information for referrals; arrange hospital admissions and surgery; schedule patients for outpatient diagnostic tests; manage recall system and file; employ procedures for handling cancellations and missed appointments.	
4. Oral and written communications—Answer and place telephone calls employing proper etiquette; manage telephone calls requiring special attention (including lab and x-ray reports, angry callers, and personal calls); instruct patients by telephone regarding emergency treatment and medications; inform patients of laboratory results; employ effective intraoffice oral communication skills (including employee supervision and patient handling); compose correspondence according to acceptable business format; type bills, statements, medical records, and other written materials, and proofread written material; manage mail; employ effective written communication skills.	
5. Records management—Manage complete patient medical records system; file records according to appropriate system (master calendars, tickler files, correspondence, financial records, physician's records, nonpatient files); transfer files; protect, store, and retain medical records according to appropriate conventions.	
6. Charts—Arrange contents of patient charts in appropriate order and perform audits for accuracy; record laboratory results and patient communication in charts; maintain confidentiality of medical records and test results (e.g., HIV, pregnancy tests); observe special regulations regarding the confidentiality of HIV results.	4
7. Transcription and dictation—Transcribe notes from dictaphone or tape recorder; transcribe notes from direct dictation.	

AMT Registered Medical Assistant (RMA) Certification Exam Topics Correlation Chart (cont.)

Exam Topics	Student Edition
8. Supplies and equipment management—Maintain inventory of medical and office supplies and equipment (reordering, order new supplies); arrange for equipment maintenance and repair, and maintain warranty/services files.	4, 19
9. Computers for medical office applications—Use computer for data entry and retrieval; use computer for word processing; use computer for billing and financial transactions; employ procedures for ensuring the integrity and confidentiality of computer-stored information.	
10. Office safety—Maintain office cleanliness and comfort; maintain office safety (maintain office safety manual and post-emergency instructions); maintain records of biohazardous waste and hazardous chemicals; know and comply with Occupational Safety and Health Act (OSHA) guidelines and regulations.	1, 4, 6
III. Clinical Medical Assisting	
A. Asepsis	
1. Terminology—Know terminology associated with asepsis.	6
2. Universal blood and body fluid precautions—Know transmission and prevention of transmission of microorganisms; know and follow OSHA guidelines for bloodborne pathogens.	6
3. Medical asepsis—Know and follow aseptic procedures when working; employ hand washing and gloving procedures.	6
4. Surgical asepsis—Know and perform surgical aseptic techniques; employ surgical hand washing and gloving procedures.	6
B. Sterilization	
1. Terminology—Know terminology associated with sterilization procedures.	6, 8, 19
2. Sanitization—Know the procedures for sanitization of various equipment found in the medical office; know the various chemicals used for sanitization.	4, 6, 19
3. Disinfection—Know procedures for disinfection of various disinfection chemicals; know the names of, and uses for, various disinfection chemicals.	4, 6, 19
4. Sterilization—Employ procedures for sterilizing items (gloves, instruments, tubing, jars, solutions, and drapes); know proper sterilization methods for items (e.g., autoclave, chemical sterilization); know the procedures for wrapping items; know the various types of wrapping materials; describe the various types of indicators.	4, 6, 19

AMT Registered Medical Assistant (RMA) Certification Exam Topics Correlation Chart (cont.)

Exam Topics	Student Edition
C. Instruments	
1. Identification—Know various instrument parts (i.e., handles, locks, teeth, and serrations); know instrument classifications; name commonly used instruments; name specialty instruments.	19
2. Usage—Know the use of each of the commonly used instruments (i.e., forceps, hemostats, scissors); know the instruments used for various types of examinations (i.e., gynecological, pediatric, neurological, and physical examinations).	
3. Care and handling—Know the procedure for care of nondisposable instruments; know the procedure for discarding disposable instruments.	19
D. Vital Signs	
1. Blood pressure—Obtain blood pressure (select proper cuff size, employ appropriate and accurate procedure); record measurement; recognize normal and abnormal blood pressure readings.	9, 10
2. Pulse—Obtain a pulse, know various locations that can be used; record pulse; recognize normal and abnormal pulse.	9
3. Respiration—Obtain a respiratory rate; record respiration; recognize normal and abnormal respiration rate.	10
4. Height and weight—Obtain height and weight; record height and weight; know terminology associated with abnormal measurements; obtain and record pediatric height and weight.	
5. Temperature—Know the types, care, and handling of thermometers; obtain temperatures via oral, rectal, and axillary methods; know normal temperature ranges for each method; record temperature; know fever classifications.	
E. Physical Examinations	
1. Problem oriented records—Obtain medical history; employ appropriate terminology and abbreviations; differentiate between subjective and objective information (describe what constitutes each); understand SOAP procedure for recording information.	4
2. Positions—Know positions used for examinations; know when to utilize each; drape patient for each examination.	
3. Methods of examination—Know methods used for physical examinations; know when to employ each method.	
4. Specialty examinations—Know procedures for pediatric examinations, including Apgar scoring, head circumference measurements, and growth charts; know procedures for gynecological and obstetric examinations, including Pap smears, breast examinations, and routine obstetric examinations; know procedures for proctological examinations, including rectal, proctoscopy, and sigmoidoscopy; know procedures for genitourinary tract examinations.	

AMT Registered Medical Assistant (RMA) Certification Exam Topics Correlation Chart (cont.)

Exam Topics	Student Edition
5. Visual acuity—Know procedures for obtaining near and far visual acuity (employ adult and pediatric charts); know procedures for obtaining color vision acuity; know normal and abnormal measurements.	
6. Allergy testing—Know procedure for performing scratch test; know procedure for performing intradermal skin test; know terminology associated with allergy specialty.	
F. Clinical Pharmacology	
1. Terminology—Know terminology associated with pharmacology; know commonly used abbreviations.	1–20
2. Injections—Know procedures for performing intramuscular, subcutaneous, intradermal, and z-tract injections; know sites and amounts used for each type; know procedure for obtaining a drug from a vial or ampule; know needle sizes and syringe types necessary for each injection type; perform calculations required for dosages, including conversion factors; prepare documentation.	3, 4, 19
3. Prescriptions—Know drug schedules and legal procedure for each; know procedures for completing prescriptions, refills, and patient documentation.	1, 2, 4
4. Drugs—Know regulation of medications, including proper record maintenance and Drug Enforcement Agency regulations; know categories, forms, and uses of drugs; know commonly used drugs; know methods of administration other than injections; rectal, topical, vaginal, sublingual, oral, and inhalation; know procedure for ear instillation, eye drops, and ointments; know drug storage requirements (i.e., narcotics, locked cabinets, refrigeration, etc.); know procedure for using *Physician's Desk Reference*®.	1–20
G. Minor Surgery	
1. Surgical supplies—Know supplies used in minor surgery, including drapes, dressings, bandages, sutures, anesthetics, and antiseptics; identify by name, and use, instruments common to office surgery.	
2. Surgical procedures—Know procedure for surgical tray preparation, including the use of sterile packs, transfer forceps, and sterile containers; know procedure for patient preoperative and postoperative skin care; handle sterile equipment using aseptic technique; identify potential contamination through personnel, moisture, and equipment handling; employ aseptic technique for hand washing and gloving; know procedures for removing all types of sutures; know dressing and bandaging procedures; know other surgical procedures; know care of equipment, skin preparation, and patient care for electrosurgery; know precautions, preparation, and patient care for laser surgery; dispose of contaminated disposable instruments.	

AMT Registered Medical Assistant (RMA) Certification Exam Topics Correlation Chart (cont.)

Exam Topics	Student Edition
H. Therapeutic Modalities	
1. Modalities—Know procedures for performing heat treatments, including hot pack, moist compress, hot water bottle, heat lamp, paraffin bath, and whirlpool bath; know procedures for applying ice pack and cold compress; know procedure for performing ultrasound treatments; know range-of-motion joint exercises.	
2. Patient instruction—Instruct patients in the use of crutches, canes, wheelchairs, etc.; instruct patients regarding therapeutic treatments at home, as directed by physician.	
I. Laboratory Procedures	
1. Safety—Employ universal blood and body fluid precautions and OSHA guidelines.	6
2. Quality control—Establish and perform quality control procedures.	4
3. Laboratory equipment—Employ proper care and use of laboratory equipment, including microscopes, centrifuges, refractometer, and glassware.	
4. Urinalysis—Know procedures for obtaining sterile, clean catch, timed, and drug screening specimens; know procedures for performing urinalysis, including physical characteristics, chemical (dipstick), and microscope preparation.	12
5. Blood—Obtain a blood specimen by venipuncture and fingerstick (including selection of proper specimen container); perform microhematocrit, hemoglobin, blood glucose (by reagent strip or Accu-Check), sedimentation rate; know procedures for proper disposal of blood products.	
6. Other specimens—Obtain a swab throat culture; obtain a stool specimen for occult blood and parasite determination; assist in obtaining cerebral spinal fluid; know procedure for obtaining sputum specimen.	6, 10, 11
7. Specimen handling—Label and handle reference laboratory specimens; complete request forms.	12
8. Records—Know appropriate record and documentation procedures.	
9. Microbiology—Identify microorganism categories; know names and growth patterns of pathogenic organisms; know procedures for obtaining laboratory specimens; know procedures for preparing slides for physician microscopic examination (i.e., wet mount).	
J. Electrocardiography	
1. Standard, 12-lead ECG—Know procedure for patient preparation, lead placement, and obtaining a 12-lead ECG; identify and eliminate artifacts; know ECG lead marking codes.	9

AMT Registered Medical Assistant (RMA) Certification Exam Topics Correlation Chart (cont.)

Exam Topics	Student Edition
2. Mounting techniques—Know procedure for mounting an ECG; identify abnormal readings for mounting.	
3. Other ECG procedures—Know procedure for obtaining a rhythm strip; identify special ECG procedures (i.e., Holter monitor, treadmill examinations, etc.).	
K. First Aid	
1. First aid procedures—Perform CPR and Heimlich maneuver; maintain a crash tray; identify first aid emergencies and associated procedures (i.e., strokes, heart attacks, fractures, animal bites, shock, asthma, poisoning, seizures, sprains, strains, burns, head injuries, lacerations, epistaxis, hemorrhages, injuries, and foreign bodies); know terminology and abbreviations associated with first aid.	
2. Legal responsibilities—Know legal responsibilities as they apply to the medical assistant (i.e., reporting, action to be taken); report emergencies as required by law.	

SCANS (Secretary's Commission on Achieving Necessary Skills) Correlation Chart

Competencies	Student Edition
I. Resources: Identifies, organizes, plans, and allocates resources	
A. Time—Selects goal-relevant activities, ranks them, allocates time, and prepares and follows schedules	
B. Money—Uses or prepares budgets, makes forecasts, keeps records, and makes adjustments to meet objectives	
C. Material and Facilities—Acquires, stores, allocates, and uses materials or space efficiently	1, 4
D. Human Resources—Assesses skills and distributes work accordingly, evaluates performance and provides feedback	
II. Interpersonal: Works with others	
A. Participates as Member of a Team—Contributes to group effort	
B. Teaches Others New Skills	5–20
C. Serves Clients/Customers—Works to satisfy customers' expectations	5–20
D. Exercises Leadership—Communicates ideas to justify position, persuades and convinces others, responsibly challenges existing procedures and policies	
E. Negotiates—Works toward agreements involving exchange of resources, resolves divergent interests	
F. Works With Diversity—Works well with men and women from diverse backgrounds	5–20
III. Information: Acquires and uses information	
A. Acquires and Evaluates Information	1–20
B. Organizes and Maintains Information	1–20
C. Interprets and Communicates Information	1–20
D. Uses Computers to Process Information	
IV. Systems: Understands complex interrelationships	
A. Understands Systems—Knows how social, organizational, and technological systems work and operates effectively with them	
B. Monitors and Corrects Performance—Distinguishes trends, predicts impacts on system operations, diagnoses deviations in systems' performance and corrects malfunctions	
C. Improves or Designs Systems—Suggest modifications to existing systems and develops new or alternative systems to improve performance	

SCANS (Secretary's Commission on Achieving Necessary Skills) Correlation Chart (cont.)

Competencies	Student Edition
V. Technology: Works with a variety of technologies	
A. Selects Technology—Chooses procedures, tools, or equipment, including computers and related technologies	
B. Applies Technology to Task—Understands overall intent and proper procedures for setup and operation of equipment	
C. Maintains and Troubleshoots Equipment—Prevents, identifies, or solves problems with equipment, including computers and other technologies	

National Health Care Skill Standards Correlation Chart

Standards	Student Edition
I. Health Care Core Standards—The industry core is a set of broad standards that serve as a foundation to occupations and functions across the health services. These standards specify the knowledge and skills that the vast majority of health care workers should have.	
A. Academic Foundation—Health care workers will know the academic subject matter required for proficiency within their area. They will use this knowledge as needed in their role.	
1. Read and write, including charts, reports, and manuals.	4
2. Perform mathematical functions.	3
3. Use health care terminology.	1–20
4. Apply knowledge of life sciences, such as biology, chemistry, physics, and human growth and development.	1–20
5. Be aware of the history of health care.	
B. Communication—Health care workers will know various communication methods to give and obtain information. They will communicate effectively, both orally and in writing.	
1. Assess others' ability to understand.	
2. Adapt communication to individual needs, including paraphrasing or translating.	5–20
3. Ask for clarification when needed.	
4. Be sensitive to multicultural and multilingual needs.	5–20
5. Use facility-specific guidelines and methods of sending and receiving information.	
6. Access and use electronically produced information.	
C. Systems—Health care workers will understand how their role fits in with their department, their setting, and the overall health care environment. They will identify how key systems relate to the services they perform and affect quality of care.	
1. Be aware of the range of services offered.	
2. Be aware of how reimbursement affects care delivery.	
3. Prevent unnecessary waste and duplication.	
4. Fully use available facility resources, such as where to find help or information.	
D. Employability Skills—Health care workers will understand how employability skills enhance their employment opportunities and job satisfaction. They will demonstrate key employability skills and will maintain and upgrade skills, as needed.	
1. Exhibit personal skills, such as attendance, time management, and individual responsibility.	
2. Maintain professional conduct and appearance.	
3. Use analytical skills to solve problems and make decisions.	3, 5–20

National Health Care Skill Standards Correlation Chart (cont.)

Standards	Student Edition
4. Adapt to changing situations.	
5. Upgrade technology skills as needed.	
6. Understand various career options and the preparation required for them.	
7. Anticipate needs of clients and coworkers.	
E. Legal Responsibilities—Health care workers will understand their legal responsibilities, limitations, and the implications of their actions within the health care delivery setting. They will perform their duties in accordance with laws, regulations, policies, and legislated rights of clients.	
1. Be aware of malpractice and liability issues.	1, 4
2. Maintain client confidentiality.	1, 4
3. Operate within scope of practice.	1, 4
4. Comply with legal requirements for documentation.	1, 4
F. Ethics—Health care workers will understand accepted ethical practices with respect to cultural, social, and ethnic differences, particularly within the health care environment. They will perform their duties within established ethical guidelines, supporting sensitive and quality health care delivery.	
1. Exhibit loyalty to fellow workers and the organization.	
2. Respect client rights and self-determination.	1, 4
3. Promote justice and equal treatment of all persons.	
4. Recognize the importance of client need over other considerations.	5–20
5. Report any activity that adversely affects the health, safety, or welfare of clients and fellow workers.	5–20
G. Safety Practices—Health care workers will be aware of the existing and potential hazards to clients, coworkers, and self. They will prevent injury or illness through safe work practices and follow health and safety policies and procedures.	
1. Use Universal Precautions to control the spread of infection.	6
2. Apply principles of body mechanics, such as proper lifting techniques.	
3. Prevent fire and electrical hazards.	
4. Use instruments and equipment as directed.	4, 19
5. Manage hazardous materials.	6
6. Follow emergency procedures and protocols.	
7. Apply pertinent regulatory guidelines, including OSHA standards.	4, 6

National Health Care Skill Standards Correlation Chart (cont.)

Standards	Student Edition
H. Interpersonal Dynamics—Health care workers will understand the role and responsibilities of individual members as part of the health care team, including their ability to promote the delivery of quality health care. They will interact effectively and sensitively with all members of the health care team.	
1. Practice team membership skills, such as cooperation, leadership, and listening.	
2. Respect cultural and religious differences of team members.	
3. Be aware of the implications of the health care hierarchy in interacting with others.	
4. Manage conflict within the work place through consideration of others' points of view.	
5. Respect inter- and intradisciplinary issues.	
II. Therapeutic/Diagnostic Core Standards—The therapeutic-diagnostic/core standards are a set of standards that apply to both therapeutic and diagnostic occupations and functions. The standards focus, for the most part, on direct client care.	
A. Health Maintenance Practices—Therapeutic and diagnostic workers will understand the fundamentals of wellness and the treatment of disease processes. They will encourage the practice of preventive health behaviors among their clients.	
1. Be knowledgeable of available preventive health screenings and examinations.	5–20
2. Explain preventive health practices, such as good nutrition and stress management.	5–20
3. Show knowledge of illness prevention.	5–20
B. Client Interaction—Therapeutic and diagnostic workers will understand how to explain planned procedures and goals to clients. They will use various explanation strategies and answer clients' questions.	
1. Determine clients' ability to understand.	5–20
2. Respond to clients' concerns and fears.	5–20
3. Use language appropriate to the situation.	5–20
4. Use facility guidelines for giving health information.	5–20
5. Respect clients' cultural differences.	5–20
C. Intrateam Communication—Therapeutic and diagnostic workers will understand how to communicate within a team. They will convey critical client information to appropriate team members in a timely manner.	
1. Observe and report unsafe environmental conditions.	6
2. Recognize unusual occurrences in treatment progress.	
3. Document and report information about changes in conditions that might introduce risk to clients or staff.	

National Health Care Skill Standards Correlation Chart (cont.)

Standards	Student Edition
D. Monitoring Client Status—Therapeutic and diagnostic workers will understand the process for monitoring client health status. They will assess health status according to respective professional standards and report results to the treatment team.	
1. Measure and report client vital signs or other indicators of health status.	
2. Record client health status according to facility protocol.	
3. Assist in determining the need for follow-up or alternative care.	
E. Client Movement—Therapeutic and diagnostic workers will understand the principles of proper body mechanics for positioning, transferring, and transporting clients. They will perform these activities efficiently and without injury to clients or self.	
1. Position client to ensure comfort.	
2. Recognize center of gravity and base of support in order to use proper lifting techniques.	
3. Utilize appropriate transport or transfer equipment.	
4. Reassure clients and inform them of what to expect during activity.	5–20

CHAPTER 1

Orientation to Medications

Objectives

- Define *pharmacology, pharmacodynamics, pharmacy, anatomy, physiology,* and *pathology.*
- List the major sources of drugs and give examples of each.
- List the six uses of drugs.
- Define drug standards and tell how they are determined.
- Explain why drug standards are necessary.
- List and describe four types of names by which drugs are known.
- Name three drug references and show how to use at least one.
- Use drug references to prepare a drug card.
- Name three major drug laws and list their main features.
- Name the federal agencies that enforce the drug laws.
- Explain why health workers must be familiar with drug laws.

Chapter Outline

Key Terms
Pharmacology
Drug Sources
Drug Uses
Drug Standards
Drug Names
Drug References
Preparing Your Own Drug Cards
Drug Legislation
You and the Law
Health Care For Today and Tomorrow
Legal and Ethical Issues
Chapter 1 Review

Teaching Strategies

- Ask students to identify the key terms they are already familiar with. Discuss the definitions of all the terms and be certain that students are clear about the meanings. Point out any similarities that may be confusing to them and tell them to memorize those words to avoid confusion later on. Ask volunteers to share their methods of learning medical key terms.
- Ask students to list the major sources of drugs and give examples of each.
- If possible, obtain a film from the library or a pharmaceutical company explaining the process of drug trials. Show the film to the class.
- Take a field trip to a pharmaceutical company in your area to observe the step-by-step process of manufacturing drugs. Ask students to summarize why, as health care workers, they should understand the drug manufacturing process. Discuss how the company followed drug legislation.
- Invite a pharmacist into class (or visit a pharmacy) to discuss the process of testing for generic drugs. Ask students why it is important they understand this process.

- Ask a pharmaceutical representative to speak to the class about how he or she can make a difference in patient care.
- Visit a local pharmacy or invite a pharmacist into class to discuss what pharmacists teach patients when they dispense a drug. Ask for print material that is sometimes given to patients. Discuss in class how this material could be beneficial or harmful to the patient.
- When students begin work in a health facility, ask them to make a list of all the drug references that are available to them in their work environment. Are the materials up-to-date? Why are up-to-date references important to the patient and the health care worker?
- Ask students to complete the Chapter 1 Review. Discuss answers, clearing up any misconceptions students may have. Review any material students had difficulty with.
- Administer and grade the Chapter 1 Test in this Instructor's Manual.
- Develop and administer a performance test for preparing a drug card.

Critical Thinking Activity

You are admitting a patient who frequently changes physicians. The patient has an unlabeled bottle of pills that she has been taking. She says that a doctor she no longer sees prescribed them for her. She does not know why she was taking the drug or the name of the drug. What should you do to determine the drug's name, action, and therapeutic purpose?

Answers to Chapter 1 Review

1. Chemical substance used in the diagnosis, treatment, cure, or prevention of a particular disease.
2. The study of drugs: sources, chemical makeup, uses, how to prepare them, and so on.
3. The structure of the body and its parts.
4. The science that deals with the functions of cells, tissues, and organs of living organisms.
5. Rules concerning the strength, quality, and purity of drugs.
6. *Physicians' Desk Reference®*, a drug reference.
7. *United States Pharmacopeia/National Formulary,* a drug reference containing the standards for official drugs.
8. Study of the changes in the body caused by disease.
9. The absorption, distribution, metabolism, and excretion of drugs.
10. Drug sources include:
    - Plants—digitalis, opium, belladonna, vitamin C, gums, oils.
    - Animals—insulin, heparin.
    - Minerals—iron, iodine, salt, calcium.
    - Synthetic drugs—*Bactrim, Septra,* biotechnology, Humulin® insulin, vaccines.
11. Drug uses:
    - Prevent diseases—vaccines.
    - Maintain health—insulin, vitamins.
    - Diagnose disease—radiopaque dye, barium.
    - Treat disease—aspirin, antihistamines.
    - Cure disease—antibiotics.
    - Prevent pregnancy—contraceptives.

12. Drug laws and agencies:
    - Pure Food and Drug Act of 1906, no agency.
    - Food, Drug, and Cosmetic Act of 1938, enforced by the FDA.
    - Controlled Substances Act of 1970, enforced by the DEA.
13. OTC drugs can be bought and sold without a prescription. Prescription drugs need a doctor's written or verbal order to be bought and sold. Controlled substances have restrictions on who can prescribe, how, and how often.

14. c 15. b 16. a 17. d 18. f 19. e 20. e
21. b 22. a 23. d 24. c

25. Janie should study the federal and state laws controlling medication administration. She should also study the nursing home's own regulations, and she should find out who is in charge so that she knows to whom questions should be addressed.
26. Answers will vary.
27. Pink.
28. About 17 (this will vary from year to year).
29. Acetaminophen.

Chapter 1 Test Answers

1. c 2. a 3. a 4. b 5. c 6. d 7. d
8. d 9. a 10. c 11. a 12. c 13. d 14. c
15. b 16. c 17. a 18. c 19. d 20. d 21. b
22. d 23. a 24. d

CHAPTER 2
Principles of Drug Action

Objectives

- State the four basic drug actions.
- Name and describe the four body processes that affect drug action.
- Identify at least 10 factors influencing drug action.
- Differentiate between systemic and local drug effects.
- State the difference between the therapeutic effect and side effects.
- Differentiate among synergism, antagonism, and potentiation.
- Explain the difference between psychological and physical drug dependence.
- List five commonly abused drugs.
- State the health worker's responsibilities with regard to adverse reactions, drug dependence, and drug abuse.

Chapter Outline

Key Terms
Pharmacokinetics
Drug Action
Factors Affecting Drug Action
Drug Effects

Adverse Reactions

Drug Dependence or Drug Abuse?

Chapter 2 Review

Teaching Strategies

- Discuss the definitions of the key terms and have the students give an example of how each term is used.
- Ask students to use a drug reference to find side effects that are not adverse reactions. This activity is more meaningful if you select a drug one of the students is taking or has recently taken.
- Obtain and show a film on drug addiction. Ask the students to summarize the difference between physical and psychological dependence.
- Make arrangements for the class to visit a community-based psychiatric hospital or clinic to observe patients who have been abusing drugs.
- Arrange for a panel discussion to include drug counselors, crisis center workers, former addicts, and alcoholics to provide the students with the opportunity to obtain firsthand knowledge from the victims of abuse.
- Ask students to attend an AA meeting and write a summary of the experience. Also ask them to bring back any literature that is available.
- Discuss the potential of drug abuse in health care workers. Discuss what is the worker's responsibility if he or she suspects a fellow health care worker to have a drug abuse situation.
- Develop a class discussion on how a health care worker might help a drug-impaired health care worker.
- Have students work in cooperative learning groups to make a display that describes the local and systemic processes of drug effects in the body.
- Ask students to explain the difference between synergism, antagonism, and potentiation.
- Divide students into two cooperative learning groups. Identify five drug categories. After group one has identified the therapeutic effects of those identified drugs and group two has identified the side effects of the same drugs, have a class discussion on the differences.
- Ask students to complete the Chapter 2 Review. Discuss answers, clearing up any misconceptions students may have. Review any material students had difficulty with.
- Administer and grade the Chapter 2 Test in this Instructor's Manual.

Critical Thinking Activity

Have each student imagine caring for a patient who started on a new drug a week ago and was given information on the side effects of that medication. The patient now says that he is experiencing all of the side effects mentioned a week ago. Ask the student to consider if the patient is suggestible or really suffering from the side effects of that drug. Ask the student what should be done.

Answers to Chapter 2 Review

1. action
2. effects
3. passage of a substance into the bloodstream from the site of administration
4. movement of drugs into cells and into spaces between cells
5. breaking down drugs into different substances that can be excreted
6. removal of waste products from the body
7. systemic

8. local
9. speeding up (stimulating), slowing down (depressing), stopping or destroying
10. replacing
11. absorption, distribution, biotransformation, excretion
12. kidneys, large intestine, lungs, milk glands
13. therapeutic and side effects
14. any three of the following: skin rashes, itchy eyes, itchy skin, wheezing, fever, nasal drainage.
15. an inactive substance that has no pharmacological effect
16. self-administration of a drug in chronically excessive amounts resulting in psychological and/or physical dependence
17. overuse or improper use of any drug
18. abnormal or peculiar response to certain drugs
19. five of the following: narcotics and opium; barbiturates, sedatives or hypnotics, and alcohol; amphetamines, cocaine, and other stimulants; LSD and other hallucinogens; marijuana
20. consult the nurse in charge
21. a condition in which the body must have a drug in order to function because it is so used to having the drug
22. a feeling of being unable to get along without a drug
23. Symptomatic and supportive.
24. Laxative, acetaminophen, aspirin, nicotine, alcohol.
25. Breathing and heart stop.
26. Shortens the time needed for symptoms to appear, potentiates the effect of the drug.
27. Drug that has the opposite effect and can reverse the overdose symptoms.
28. Dose of a drug that is too large for the patient's size, age, or physical condition.

29. —	30. √	31. —	32. √	33. √
34. √	35. —	36. —	37. √	38. √
39. √	40. √	41. √	42. √	43. √
44. —	45. √	46. —	47. —	

48. tolerance	49. cumulative effect
50. potentiation (or synergism)	51. drug dependence
52. antagonism	53. idiosyncrasy
54. drug allergy	55. drug interaction

56. overdose
57. Adverse Event Report
58. in back of *PDR*® and is allowed to be copied
59. Vaccine Adverse Event Reporting System
60. to compare it with the patient's history and the conditions at hand

Chapter 2 Test Answers

1. a	2. c	3. a	4. b	5. d	6. c	7. c
8. b	9. b	10. d	11. c	12. d	13. d	14. a
15. b	16. a	17. b	18. a	19. c	20. d	21. a
22. c	23. b	24. f	25. e			

CHAPTER 3

Measurement and Dosage Calculation

Objectives

- Write and define the abbreviations for units of measurement in the metric, apothecary, and household systems.
- State the most common equivalents among apothecary, metric, and household measures and use a conversion table to find less common equivalents.
- Convert grams to milligrams and vice versa.
- Convert milliliters to teaspoons and vice versa.
- Calculate the number of tablets or capsules to give when the available dose differs from the ordered dose.
- Calculate doses using a procedure for converting between different units of measurement.
- Calculate an adult's dose of medication.
- Calculate a child's dose of medication.
- Calculate drops per minute for IV therapy.

Chapter Outline

Key Terms
Math Review: Fractions
Systems of Measurement
Converting Among Measurement Systems
Dosage Calculation
Health Care for Today and Tomorrow
Legal and Ethical Issues
Chapter 3 Review

Teaching Strategies

- Discuss the meanings of the key terms. Be sure students understand all of the terms before proceeding.
- Ask students to make cards, posters, flashcards, or displays that can be used to help them learn the abbreviations and equivalents found in Tables 3-1 through 3-7 in the text.
- Encourage students to share their learning tools and to use them as needed.
- Calculate dose using a procedure for converting between different units of measurement.
- Set up stations in the lab to resemble a patient room, a medicine room, and an emergency cart that includes IV equipment. At each station arrange appropriate forms of medications with dosage labels. Make medicine cards that require students to calculate the proper dosage. On the back of the cards place the answers. Have students in groups or individually go to each station and calculate the various dosages. Ask them to repeat any of the calculations they missed.
- Ask students to complete the Chapter 3 Review. Discuss answers, clearing up any misconceptions students may have. Review any material students had difficulty with.
- Administer and grade the Chapter 3 Test in this Instructor's Manual.

Critical Thinking Activity

Calculate a dose of medication to be administered to a patient intramuscularly. When you go to give the medication, the patient says the syringe you are using is too big and contains more medicine than usual. What should you do?

Answers to Chapter 3 Review

1. The different amounts of a drug that will produce therapeutic effects but not serious side effects or toxicity.
2. Basic unit of weight in the apothecary system.
3. A decimal system of measurement in which the basic unit of length is the meter, the basic unit of volume is the liter, and the basic unit of weight is the gram.
4. Basic unit of volume in the apothecary system.
5. Basic unit of volume in the metric system.
6. Basic unit of length in the metric system.
7. A mathematical way of talking about an amount that is part of a whole or a ratio between two numbers.
8. One-hundredth of a meter.
9. One-thousandth of a liter, the same as a cubic centimeter.

10. Min	11. gr	12. dr	13. fldr
14. oz	15. gt	16. pt	17. T, tbsp
18. lb	19. mg	20. ml	21. cc, cm^3
22. L, l	23. g, gm	24. 4 fluidrams	25. 1½ grains
26. 2 minims	27. 9 fluidrams	28. one	29. one
30. 15	31. 1	32. 60	33. 1000
34. one	35. 500	36. one	37. $\frac{1}{2}$
38. $\frac{1}{3}$	39. $\frac{3}{4}$	40. $\frac{3}{4}$	41. $\frac{1}{4}$
42. $\frac{5}{9}$	43. $2\frac{2}{3}$	44. $2\frac{1}{2}$	45. $1\frac{5}{12}$
46. $2\frac{3}{4}$	47. $4\frac{1}{2}$	48. $22\frac{2}{3}$	49. $3\frac{1}{2}$
50. $5\frac{2}{5}$	51. $\frac{3}{100}$	52. $1\frac{1}{4}$	53. $4\frac{1}{6}$ gr
54. $\frac{5}{12}$	55. $1\frac{11}{24}$	56. 180 mg	57. $\frac{3}{4}$
58. $\frac{1}{180}$	59. $1\frac{1}{8}$	60. 600	61. 0.5
62. 0.25	63. 0.75	64. 0.25	65. 0.023
66. 0.333	67. 0.667	68. 0.6	69. 0.89
70. 3.75	71. $\frac{3}{4}$	72. $1\frac{1}{2}$	73. $\frac{1}{200}$
74. $\frac{1}{5}$	75. $5\frac{2}{3}$	76. $\frac{3}{8}$	77. 4.5
78. 0.045	79. 0.3	80. 0.45	81. 0.275
82. 3	83. 100	84. 30	85. 0.325
86. 3	87. 2500	88. 125	89. 1.2
90. 0.005	91. 36.3°	92. 37.2°	93. 37.8°
94. 38.8°	95. 38.9°	96. 40°	97. 95.8°
98. 99.3°	99. 102.6°	100. 104°	101. 105.6°
102. 107.6°	103. $\frac{1}{600}$	104. $\frac{1}{120}$	105. 1
106. $\frac{1}{15}$	107. $2\frac{1}{2}$	108. 300	109. 15
110. 0.5	111. $2\frac{1}{2}$ $(\frac{250}{100} = 2\frac{1}{2})$	112. $\frac{1}{4}\left(\frac{\frac{5}{4}}{5} = \frac{5}{4} \times \frac{1}{5}\right)$	
113. 3 $(\frac{75}{25} = 3)$	114. 4 $(\frac{400,000}{100,000} = 4)$		
115. 2 $(\frac{50}{25} = 2)$	116. $\frac{1}{2}\left(\frac{\frac{1}{4}}{\frac{1}{2}} = \frac{1}{4} \times \frac{2}{1} = \frac{1}{2}\right)$		

117. $2\left(\frac{15}{\frac{15}{2}} = 15 \times \frac{2}{15} = 2\right)$

118. 1

119. 1

120. $\frac{11}{2}$

121. 3

122. a. 48 tsp $\left(\begin{array}{l}\text{(8 fl oz contains 16T;}\\ \text{to get teaspoons, multiply by 3)}\\ \text{(or } 16\cancel{T} \times \frac{3\text{ tsp}}{1\cancel{T}} = 48\text{ tsp)}\end{array}\right)$

b. 48 days

123. 7.3 mg $\left(11\ \cancel{\text{mos}} \times \frac{\overset{2}{\cancel{100}}\text{ mg}}{\underset{3}{\cancel{150}}\ \cancel{\text{mos}}} = \frac{22\text{ mg}}{3} = 7.3\text{ mg}\right)$

124. 23 mg $\left(34\ \cancel{\text{lb}} \times \frac{\overset{2}{\cancel{100}}\text{ mg}}{\underset{3}{\cancel{150}}\ \cancel{\text{lb}}} = \frac{68\text{ mg}}{3} = 22\tfrac{2}{3}\text{ mg, or about 23 mg}\right)$

125. 80 mg $\left(10\text{ yr} = 120\text{ mos; } 120\ \cancel{\text{mos}} \times \frac{\overset{2}{\cancel{100}}\text{ mg}}{\underset{3}{\cancel{150}}\ \cancel{\text{mos}}} = \frac{240}{3}\text{ mg} = 80\text{ mg}\right)$

126. 100 mg (Anyone over 12½ years old is considered an adult.)

127. 25 gtt/minute $\left(\frac{\overset{100}{\cancel{500}}\ \cancel{\text{cc}}}{\underset{1}{\cancel{5}}\ \cancel{\text{hour}}} \times \frac{\overset{1}{\cancel{15}}\text{ gtt}}{1\ \cancel{\text{cc}}} \times \frac{1\ \cancel{\text{hour}}}{\underset{4}{\cancel{60}}\text{ minutes}} = \frac{100}{4}\text{ or 25 gtt/minute}\right)$

128. 33 gtt/minute $\left(\frac{\overset{100}{\cancel{500}}\ \cancel{\text{cc}}}{\underset{1}{\cancel{5}}\ \cancel{\text{hour}}} \times \frac{\overset{1}{\cancel{20}}\text{ gtt}}{1\ \cancel{\text{cc}}} \times \frac{1\ \cancel{\text{hour}}}{\underset{3}{\cancel{60}}\text{ minutes}} = \frac{100}{3}\text{ or 33 gtt/minute}\right)$

129. 16 gtt/minute $\left(\frac{\overset{250}{\cancel{1500}}\ \cancel{\text{ml}}}{\underset{4}{\cancel{24}}\ \cancel{\text{hour}}} \times \frac{\overset{1}{\cancel{15}}\text{ gtt}}{1\ \cancel{\text{cc}}} \times \frac{1\ \cancel{\text{hour}}}{\underset{4}{\cancel{60}}\text{ minutes}} = \frac{250}{16}\text{ or 15.6} = 16\text{ gtt/minute}\right)$

130. 25 gtt/minute $\left(\frac{\overset{100}{\cancel{2000}}\ \cancel{\text{cc}}}{\underset{1}{\cancel{20}}\ \cancel{\text{hour}}} \times \frac{\overset{1}{\cancel{15}}\text{ gtt}}{1\ \cancel{\text{ml}}} \times \frac{1\ \cancel{\text{hour}}}{\underset{4}{\cancel{60}}\text{ minutes}} = \frac{100}{4}\text{ or 25 gtt/minute}\right)$

Chapter 3 Test Answers

1. b	2. a	3. d	4. d	5. b	6. a	7. d
8. a	9. c	10. c	11. b	12. d	13. c	14. a
15. c	16. b	17. b	18. a	19. b	20. d	21. d
22. d	23. b	24. b	25. d	26. a	27. c	

28. 25 gtt/min

29. 40 micro gtt/min

CHAPTER 4
Medication Therapy

Objectives

- List the various forms of medication, ranging from liquids to solids.
- List and describe the routes for administering medications.
- Tell who is allowed to give medications by the parenteral route.
- Give the meaning of abbreviations for medication forms, routes, administration times, and general medical abbreviations.
- Use the military clock.
- Name the parts of a medication order.
- Identify single-dose and multiple-dose packaging of drugs.
- Outline the use of the Kardex, medicine card, and medication record to communicate medication orders.
- Set up medications following proper procedure.
- State the rules for giving medications and explain each one.
- Describe the problem-oriented medical record and the subjective–objectives–assessment–plan method of charting.
- Demonstrate accurate, complete, and organized charting.

Chapter Outline

Key Terms
Forms of Medication
Routes of Administration
The Medication Order
Types of Drug Orders
Questioning a Medication Order
Standard Medical Abbreviations
Ordering Drugs From the Pharmacy
Drug Packaging
Storage and Disposal of Drugs
Keeping Track of Medication Orders
Setting Up Medications
The Five Rights: Rules for Giving Medications
Charting Medications
The POMR
Principles of Charting
Chapter 4 Review

Teaching Strategies

- Discuss the meaning of key terms. Be sure students understand all of the terms before proceeding.
- Ask the Nursing State Board or the State Department of Education to send a representative to your class to discuss the procedures that can be performed by the various members of the health care team. Focus on RNs, LPNs, Medication Assistants, and Medical Assistants.

- Ask students who are employed (in a health care facility) to research the policies of their workplace in regard to who is allowed to administer medications, who is allowed to administer p.r.n. or parenteral medications, and who can chart and count narcotics.
- Obtain a film relating to medication therapy and show it to your class. Ask students to summarize the film and analyze its effectiveness in writing.
- Make arrangements for the class (as a group or individuals) to visit the computer lab and see a demonstration on computer use in health care. If this is not possible, ask students to visit a doctor's office or a clinic (with an appointment) to interview the office staff about the use of computers. Ask students to summarize what they learned in writing.
- Obtain samples of various forms of medications from a local pharmacist, doctor, or pharmaceutical representative. Display these in class. Ask students to identify the various forms.
- Ask students to work in four cooperative learning groups. Assign each group one of the following: Table 4-1, Table 4-2, Table 4-3, Table 4-4. Ask each group to make a chart, flashcards, or individual cards that can be used to learn the medical abbreviations. Make the "projects" available to students who want to use the devices to learn the abbreviations.
- Have students individually or in cooperative learning groups make a display of all the routes of medication administration. Tell them they can use whatever resources they can locate such as books, magazines, journals, lab equipment, catalogs, etc.
- Obtain a film relating to routine responsibilities, such as the "five rights" rule. Show the film to the class. Ask students to summarize the film in writing and to discuss its benefits.
- Make copies of a controlled substances proof-of-use record, pharmacy requisitions, a medication error form, and several different charting forms including some that make use of computers. Have students practice completing them. Then have students share forms to critique them. Discuss any problem areas.
- Have students practice the procedures listed as competencies for this chapter.
- Ask students to complete the Chapter 4 Review. Discuss answers, clearing up any misconceptions students may have. Review any material students had difficulty with.
- Administer and grade the Chapter 4 Test in this Instructor's Manual.

Answers to Chapter 4 Review

1. The ingredient in a product that produces the therapeutic effect.
2. Rinsing a body cavity with water or other solutions.
3. Administering drugs by way of droplets or mist that is breathed in.
4. Placing drops of liquid into the eyes, ears, nose, or some other body cavity.
5. Patient who is not hospitalized or institutionalized; a walk-in (or ambulatory) patient.
6. A form for writing out medication orders, located in the patient's chart.
7. Drug order in which the ordered drug is administered until a discontinuation order is written or a specified termination date is reached.
8. Drug order that outlines a specific patient condition in which a certain drug is to be administered.
9. Order for a drug to be given when a patient needs it.
10. Drug order carried out immediately and only once.

11. f 12. e 13. g 14. d 15. h 16. c 17. i

18. b 19. k 20. j 21. a 22. e 23. f 24. c
25. g 26. d 27. b 28. a 29. h 30. e 31. b
32. c 33. f 34. a 35. g 36. d

37. Extract 38. Syrup 39. Tincture
40. Suppository 41. Spirit 42. Fluidextract
43. Capsule 44. Elixir 45. Tablet
46. Solution 47. Suspension

48. Pleasant-tasting tablet made to dissolve in the mouth for a local effect.
49. Drug held in a base such as cocoa butter that melts at body temperature; designed for insertion in the vagina, rectum, or urethra.
50. Capsule containing multiple doses of medicine that are released gradually for a sustained effect.
51. Tablet with a groove down the middle for easy dividing.
52. medicine dropper or medicine glass
53. a dark place
54. alcohol
55. shaken
56. solution
57. suspension
58. enteric
59. liniments
60. rectum, vagina, urethra
61. alcohol
62. delayed-release or timed-release
63. elderly as well as young
64. added ingredients
65. food or drink
66. topical
67. parenteral
68. sterile
69. 0700 hours
70. 11:00 A.M.
71. 1:30 P.M.
72. 1400 hours
73. 8:00 P.M.
74. If you question a medication order, ask the doctor or the nurse in charge to explain the reasons for the order.
75. Physician's assistants and nurse practitioners.
76. Do not dissolve the contents of a delayed-release capsule in food or drink; this action could cause an overdose.
77. Patient's full name, date of the order, drug name, dosage, time and frequency, route of administration, signature of physician.
78. *Darvon* capsules, 65 mg every 4 hours as necessary for pain.
79. Phenobarbital elixir, 1 teaspoon (20 mg) at bedtime.
80. *Keflex* 250-mg capsules every 6 hours orally.
81. *Lotrimin* 1 percent cream twice a day for 2 weeks.
82. *Bacitracin* ophthalmic ointment in the right eye three times a day for conjunctivitis.
83. Propantheline bromide tablets, 15 mg before meals.
84. Heparin 5000 units intravenously immediately.
85. Acetaminophen 120-mg rectal suppository four times a day.

86. e 87. a 88. b 89. d 90. c 91. One

92. More than one
93. Controlled substances
94. Narcotics, barbiturates, amphetamines, hallucinogens, etc.
95. In a locked cabinet.

96. There is less chance of error because no mixing, pouring, or handling of drugs is needed. Unused doses can be returned to the pharmacy for credit.
97. In a labeled cabinet separate from the drugs for internal use.
98. Use a knife edge.
99. Right patient, right drug, right dose, right time, right route
100. Give medication from labeled containers. Read the label three times.
101. It serves as a means of communication among members of the health care team. It is a legal document, an official record of health care given. It is used for research, teaching, and evaluation of health facilities.
102. Charting Subjective comments of the patient, Objective tests of the patient's condition, the health care worker's Assessment of the problem, and a Plan of action.
103. This depends on the agency. One way is to cross out the scheduled time and initial it.
104. This depends on the agency. One way is to circle the scheduled time and initial it.

Chapter 4 Test Answers

1. b	2. d	3. c	4. a	5. b	6. a	7. c
8. d	9. d	10. c	11. a	12. b	13. c	14. a
15. d	16. d	17. c	18. b	19. d	20. d	21. d
22. b	23. c	24. b	25. c	26. b	27. d	28. a
29. b	30. d	31. a	32. c	33. d	34. b	35. a
36. d	37. c	38. b	39. a	40. a	41. d	42. a
43. b	44. b	45. b	46. a	47. d	48. b	49. c
50. a	51. c	52. c	53. d	54. c	55. b	56. c

For questions 57 through 60, see accompanying nurses' notes and medication record or a correctly filled-out form used by your agency. Slight differences in wording and format are acceptable, but be sure the following information is charted properly:

Nurses' notes:

Date

Time

Name of drug

Reason for missed medication (57 and 58)

No lines skipped

Name and title included

Errors (if any) crossed out, initialed, and rewritten

Medication record:

Missed medications circled and initialed (57 and 58) or the procedures used by your agency

P.r.n. medications charted in proper columns according to dates

All entries initialed

Signature added at bottom of page

NURSES' NOTES

Family Name	First Name	Attending Physician	Room No.	Hosp. No.
THEISS,	CAROL	DR. MEESE	124	54-783

Date	Time	REMARKS - TREATMENT	Nurses' Signature	
4/30/xx	1700	Dilantin not given. Pt. in PT. Reported to nurse in charge.	Your Name title	(57)
4/30/xx	1800	Refused chloromycetin. Stated it caused burning sensation in eyes. Reported to nurse in charge.	Your Name title	(58)
5/1/xx	1300	Tylenol gr X given for headache.	Your Name title	(59)
5/2/xx	2000	MOM 30ml given for constipation.	Your Name title	(60)

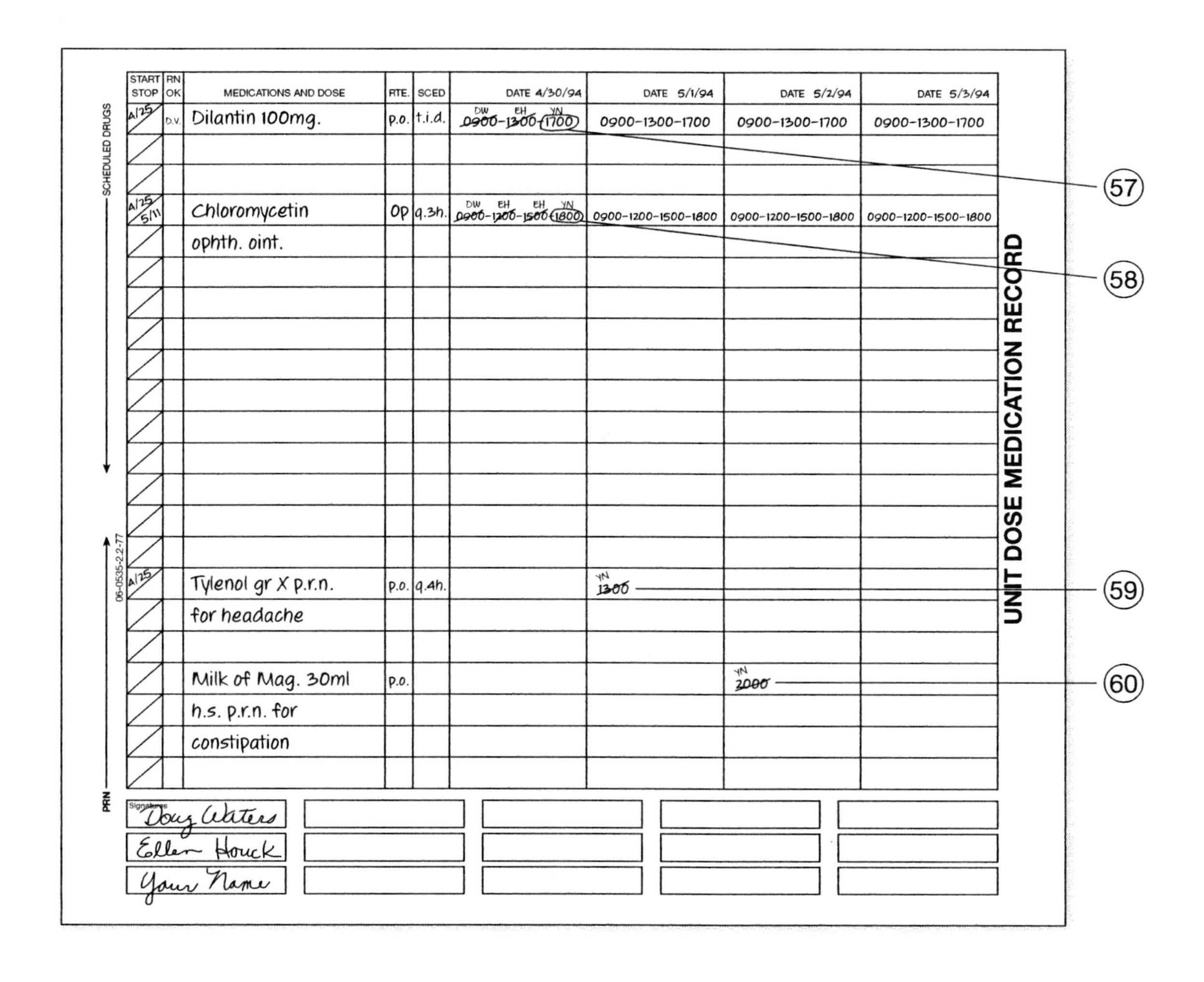

UNIT DOSE MEDICATION RECORD

START STOP	RN OK	MEDICATIONS AND DOSE	RTE.	SCED	DATE 4/30/94	DATE 5/1/94	DATE 5/2/94	DATE 5/3/94	
4/25	D.V.	Dilantin 100mg.	p.o.	t.i.d.	DW EH YN 0900-1300-(1700)	0900-1300-1700	0900-1300-1700	0900-1300-1700	(57)
4/25 5/11		Chloromycetin ophth. oint.	Op	q.3h.	DW EH EH YN 0900-1200-1500-(1800)	0900-1200-1500-1800	0900-1200-1500-1800	0900-1200-1500-1800	(58)
4/25		Tylenol gr X p.r.n. for headache	p.o.	q.4h.		YN 1300			(59)
		Milk of Mag. 30ml h.s. p.r.n. for constipation	p.o.				YN 2000		(60)

SCHEDULED DRUGS

PRN

06-0535-2-2-77

Signatures: Doug Waters, Ellen Houck, Your Name

CHAPTER 5

Vitamins, Minerals, and Herbs

Objectives

- Differentiate among the fat-soluble and water-soluble vitamins, macrominerals, and microminerals.
- Name the various vitamins and minerals.
- List the function of each vitamin and mineral.
- State the recommended daily allowance for the major vitamins and minerals.
- Identify at least two food sources of each vitamin and mineral.
- Recognize deficiency symptoms of each vitamin and mineral.
- Describe the symptoms resulting from taking large amounts of vitamins over a period of time.
- Recognize symptoms associated with elevated levels of certain minerals in the body.
- Outline the treatment for conditions resulting from too much or not enough vitamins and minerals in the body.
- Discuss the importance of patient education in the appropriate use of vitamin and mineral supplementation.
- Describe at least four herbal supplements and their uses.
- Describe the potential danger of at least four herbal remedies.

Chapter Outline

Key Terms
Recommended Daily Allowance (RDA)
Vitamins
Minerals
Electrolytes
Herbs
Health Care for Today and Tomorrow
Legal and Ethical Issues
Chapter 5 Review

Teaching Strategies

- Ask students to demonstrate their knowledge of key terms.
- Obtain and show a film on vitamins and minerals. Make sure it includes the functions, food sources, and RDA symptoms of deficiency and excess states.
- Divide students into 4 equal learning groups. Have group 1 work on the functions for each vitamin, group 2 on the food sources and RDA for each vitamin, group 3 on the symptoms of deficiency for each vitamin, and group 4 on the symptoms of excess for each vitamin. Have each group prepare a poster and present their findings to the whole class.
- Ask a dietitian to come to the class and discuss the importance of vitamins and minerals in the diet and how a hospital or community setting serving meals ensures the required RDAs.
- Ask a representative from a "health food" store to come to the class and discuss herbs.

- Arrange for the class to visit a hospital kitchen to observe how patient meals are prepared.
- Ask students to complete the Chapter 5 Review. Discuss answers, clearing up any misconceptions students may have. Review any material students had difficulty with.
- Administer and grade the Chapter 5 Test in this Instructor's Manual.

Critical Thinking Activities

1. An 80-year-old patient lives alone since the death of his wife and is proud that he prepares his own meals. His typical diet includes:

   Breakfast—egg, toast, jelly, coffee

   Lunch—lunch meat sandwich, potato chips, tea

   Dinner—canned stew or hash, coffee

   He avoids buying fresh fruits and vegetables because he says they spoil before he can use them.

   a. Discuss how this diet is deficient in the various vitamins and minerals.

   b. Develop a plan to incorporate fruits and vegetables in his diet.

2. A 30-year-old woman is in the hospital after breaking her leg skiing. She tells you that she is afraid she broke her leg because she has osteoporosis. She tells you that both her grandmothers have osteoporosis. Think of all the ways you can help this patient.

Answers to Chapter 5 Review

1. d 2. e 3. b 4. a 5. c

6. RDA 7. trace elements 8. USDA 9. B complex and C

10. fortified milk, whole milk products, green leafy vegetables, yellow fruits and vegetables, fish, liver oil, and sunlight

11. A, D, E, K 12. potassium 13. d 14. c 15. b 16. a

17. c 18. a 19. d 20. b 21. c 22. a 23. d

24. b 25. Vitamin B_1 26. Vitamin C 27. Vitamin A

28. Calcium 29. Iodine

30–31. Answers will vary depending on the edition of the *PDR*® or drug reference book used.

Chapter 5 Test Answers

1. c	2. a	3. d	4. a	5. c	6.a	7. c
8. b	9. b	10. a	11. d	12. a	13. c	14. b
15. b	16. d	17. d	18. a	19. c	20. b	21. d
22. a	23. b	24. d	25. c	26. c		

CHAPTER 6
Antibiotics and Antifungals

Objectives

- Differentiate between the external and internal immune systems.
- Explain why infection is more dangerous in a hospital or long-term care unit than elsewhere.
- State the two main actions of antibiotics and microorganisms.

- Explain why drug resistance, drug sensitivity, and superinfection are important concerns in antibiotic drug therapy.
- Name at least two problems that may arise in giving penicillin.
- List the most common uses of sulfonamides and aminoglycosides.
- Outline the importance of patient education with each of the various types of antibiotics (penicillins, cephalosporins, tetracyclines, macrolides, aminoglycosides, sulfonamides, and quinolones).
- Describe the correct procedure for hand washing before and after giving medications.
- Describe the correct procedure for administering a medication to a patient in isolation.
- State three primary ways a health care worker can be exposed to hepatitis B virus and human immunodeficiency virus.
- Explain standard, airborne, droplet, and contact precautions.

Chapter Outline

Key Terms
Infection and Immunity
Antibiotic Drugs
Antifungal Drugs
Antiviral Drugs
Isolation Procedures
Universal Blood and Body Fluid Precautions
Health Care for Today and Tomorrow
Legal and Ethical Issues
Chapter 6 Review

Teaching Strategies

- Discuss definitions of the key terms.
- Have the students brainstorm a list of terms used for "germ."
- Asks students to explain the concept of immunization. For whom is it most important? (Consider the increase in TB.)
- Ask students to refer to the Representative Drugs table at the end of the chapter. Discuss ways in which this resource will be helpful. Ask students if they have any difficulty reading it. If so, take time to answer their questions.
- Have the students use one or more drug resources to look up two or three penicillin G products. Ask them to list the most common infections each product is used for.
- If possible, obtain a medical ID bracelet. Discuss the kinds of information commonly printed on the bracelet.
- Discuss answers students may give to patients who ask why the doctor replaced one antibiotic with another after a week of therapy. (Consider the culture, sensitivity testing, and broad- versus narrow-spectrum antibiotics.)
- Ask students to refer to Table 6-1 and match as many diseases as possible from memory to an antibiotic category from Table 6-2.
- Ask students to work in cooperative learning groups to develop visuals showing the universal blood and body fluid precautions. Ask groups to critique the various presentations.
- Have the students work in cooperative learning groups to develop charts illustrating standard, airborne, droplet, and contact precautions. Ask them to cover the criteria for diseases under each category, and the barrier protection to be used for each.

- In the lab have students set up an isolation patient room. Have students practice administering medications to an isolation patient. Monitor their work. Develop a checklist from Practice Procedure 6-1 (found in the text) to use in your assessment.
- Ask students to complete the Chapter 6 Review. Discuss answers, clearing up any misconceptions students may have. Review any material students had difficulty with.
- Administer and grade the Chapter 6 Test in this Instructor's Manual.

Critical Thinking Activity

You are admitting a patient for major surgery. You notice the patient has a productive cough and says it has been a problem for 6 weeks with blood in the sputum. The patient says a family member was recently diagnosed with TB. What should you do?

Answers to Chapter 6 Review

1. Substance produced in the body to kill specific microorganisms.
2. Injection or vaccination to stimulate antibody formation against a certain microorganism.
3. Harmful microorganism, one that can cause infection.
4. Ability to inhibit growth of microorganisms.
5. Ability to kill microorganisms.
6. Symptoms relating to anaphylaxis.
7. Enzyme produced by microbes that makes them resistant to penicillin.
8. By killing microorganisms directly and by slowing the growth of microorganisms.
9. There is a risk of nerve damage that can cause deafness; the kidneys may also be damaged.
10. Macrolides.
11. The results of a Gram stain determine the choice of an antibiotic that will be most effective for a specific pathogen.
12. Isolation procedures protect the patient from microorganisms that health care workers are carrying and protect health care workers from microorganisms that the patient is carrying.
13. Strict, respiratory, and reverse (protective).

14. d 15. a 16. b 17. e 18. c 19. g 20. f

21. c 22. f 23. d 24. a 25. b 26. e

27. Infections in hospitals are dangerous because drug-resistant microorganisms that live in some health facilities cannot be killed by antibiotics. In hospitals, a large number of at-risk patients are gathered into one place. Microorganisms easily attack patients with skin wounds and lowered resistance. Medical staff can carry microorganisms from patient to patient as they work.
28. Through mucous membranes, through nonintact skin, by needlesticks.
29. Allergic reaction; superinfection; some penicillins are poorly absorbed by the oral route and/or excreted quickly; microbes develop resistance by secreting penicillinase.
30. The patient is probably allergic to penicillin and is going into anaphylactic shock. You should get emergency help immediately.
31. Antacids and dairy products prevent the proper absorption of tetracyclines from the gastrointestinal tract.

32. Secretions from the nose and mouth; secretions coughed up from lungs; feces or anything touched by feces; drainage from wounds; infected blood.

33–34. Answers will vary depending on the drug reference book or edition of the *PDR*® that is used.

Chapter 6 Test Answers

1. a	2. d	3. a	4. a	5. c	6. c	7. b
8. b	9. d	10. a	11. a	12. d	13. b	14. c
15. a	16. d	17. d	18. b	19. b	20. c	21. a
22. c	23. b	24. d	25. d	26. d	27. h	28. e
29. b	30. a	31. c	32. d	33. i	34. g	35. f

CHAPTER 7

Drugs for the Eye and Ear

Objectives

- Identify the external parts of the eye and ear.
- Describe the major disorders of the eye and ear for which medications are given.
- Describe the actions and give examples of the following drug groups: miotics, carbonic anhydrase inhibitors, beta-adrenergic blocking agents, eye antibiotics, mydriatics, and ear antibiotics.
- Follow general instructions for administering eye and ear medications.
- Follow proper procedures for instilling eyedrops, eye ointment, and ear drops.

Chapter Outline

Key Terms
Structure and Function of the Eye
Eye Disorders
Structure and Function of the Ear
Ear Disorders
Drug Therapy for Ear Disorders
Health Care for Today and Tomorrow
Legal and Ethical Issues
Chapter 7 Review

Teaching Strategies

- Discuss the meaning of the key terms. Be sure students understand all of the terms before proceeding.
- Ask students to make flashcards with key terms on one side and definitions on the opposite side. Devote a portion of a class period to having students take turns holding up a word and having a classmate give the definition.
- Show a film covering the basic anatomy of the eye and ear.
- Demonstrate the administration of eyedrops, eye ointment, and ear drops. Emphasize the importance of gloves to protect against drainage and contact with patient's body fluids.
- Arrange for a lab experience in which each student has the opportunity to do a return demonstration of the administration of eyedrops, eye ointment, and ear drops. Develop a checklist from Practice Procedure 7-1 and 7-2 (found in the text).

- If available, reserve the eye and ear structures from the health science department at your school or hand out an illustration of the structures covered in the film.
- Arrange for an ear and eye physician to visit the class and speak to students about the care of patients with disorders of the eye and ear.
- Ask students to complete the Chapter 7 Review. Discuss answers and review any material students had difficulty with.
- Administer and grade the Chapter 7 Test in this Instructor's Manual.

Critical Thinking Activities

1. You are discharging an elderly patient who is vision impaired and needs instructions on the daily administration of antiglaucoma ophthalmic drops. Develop a plan to teach the patient how to administer the drops.
2. A mother asks you how to administer antibiotic drops to her baby and if it is safe. What should you tell her?

Answers to Chapter 7 Review

1. e 2. b 3. c 4. d 5. a 6. f
7. Pertaining to hearing or sound.
8. Dizziness.
9. Pertaining to the ear.
10. Pertaining to the eye or sight.
11. Ringing in the ears.
12. Double vision.
13. malleus, incus, stapes
14. eyelid
15. eustachian tube
16. Constricts the pupil and increases aqueous humor outflow.
17. Dilates the pupil.
18. b 19. e 20. d 21. c 22. a
23. blurriness
24. cleaned and dried
25. warmed
26. "Sterile—for Ophthalmic Use"
27. Keep objects out of ears; avoid environmental noise; get all immunizations; report any vertigo, nausea, or vomiting; report mouth breathing.
28. See Table 7-1, Effects of Aging on Visual Structures
29. External otitis
30. Cerumen
31. Glaucoma
32. Conjunctivitis

33–34. Answers will vary depending on the edition of the *PDR*® used.

Chapter 7 Test Answers

1. b	2. a	3. d	4. a	5. c	6. d	7. b
8. c	9. a	10. d	11. d	12. b	13. d	14. a
15. c	16. a	17. F	18. F	19. F	20. T	21. T
22. F	23. F	24. T	25. F			

CHAPTER 8

Drugs for the Skin

Objectives

- Name the two layers of skin tissue and describe the structure of each.
- List the main functions of the integumentary system.
- Name the secretions of the sebaceous and sudoriferous glands.
- State the normal body temperature.
- Explain the process of inflammation.
- List and define the common symptoms of skin disorders.
- Describe the major skin disorders.
- State the actions and give examples of the following topical medication categories: keratolytics, protectives, astringents, antipruritics, topical corticosteroids, vasoconstrictor/venous insufficiency treatments, antiseptics, topical anesthetics, miticides, and transdermal patches.
- List five ways of increasing absorption of drugs into the skin layers.
- Follow general instructions for administering topical medications to the skin (psychological support, preparing the patient, applying bandages, etc.).
- Follow the correct procedures for applying topical creams, lotions, liniments, ointments, and aerosol sprays.

Chapter Outline

Key Terms
Integumentary System
Skin Disorders
Topical Medications
General Instructions for Medicating the Skin
Health Care for Today and Tomorrow
Legal and Ethical Issues
Chapter 8 Review

Teaching Strategies

- Discuss definitions of key terms. Be sure students understand all the terms before proceeding.
- Obtain and show a film about skin disorders. Ask students to make a list of common symptoms.
- Invite a dermatologist to speak to the class and show slides of as many skin disorders as possible. Ask about the most common OTC medications used in the office, as well as the most commonly used prescription drugs. Have students summarize the visit by listing all the disorders and drugs mentioned by the speaker.
- Ask a plastic surgeon to visit the class and speak to the students about burn patients, showing slides of first-, second-, and-third degree burns. Encourage dialogue between the physician and the students about the type of person who can care for a burn patient or work with a burn patient in the many types of therapy that will usually be necessary. (Include skin medications.)
- Make arrangements for the students either as a group or individually to visit a burn unit at a hospital. Do the caregivers appear to have the characteristics mentioned by the physician above? Why or why not?

- Assign each student a drug category from the Representative Drugs table in the text and ask them to prepare a patient case study. If they are working in a health care facility, they can select a patient they are caring for; if not, they will need to do some library research. Point out that students are encouraged to work in health care while they are completing this program. Some assignments will be directly related to work experiences.
- Ask students to bring to class the sunscreen they usually use. Divide them into cooperative learning groups and have them compare the various sunscreens. Who is most likely to have proper protection from the sun? Why is this so? What percent of the class is using this type of sunscreen? What percent will change to this type? What should they teach patients about sunscreen? What resources are available?
- In the lab, display as many topical medications as possible (creams, lotions, liniments, ointments, aerosol sprays, foams, beads, and paste). Have students practice applying these medications using Practice Procedure 8-1. Develop a checklist from the Practice Procedure to use in your assessment.
- Using the Representative Drugs table, ask students to summarize the "special instructions" column and the "side effects and adverse reactions" column in regard to administering these medications and teaching patients about them.
- Ask students to complete the Chapter 8 Review. Discuss answers, clearing up any misconceptions students may have. Review any material students had difficulty with.
- Administer and grade the Chapter 8 Test in this Instructor's Manual.

Critical Thinking Activities

1. Develop a teaching plan for the mother of a young child diagnosed with head lice. Include an emphasis on how to prevent contaminating others and preventing future episodes.
2. Develop a teaching plan on how to prevent burns.

Answers to Chapter 8 Review

1. a 2. f 3. e 4. b 5. d 6. c
7. Itching 8. Redness 9. Swelling
10. Protein contained in cells of the epidermis, nails, and hair.
11. Organism that lives on or in another organism.
12. Skin condition caused by pores being plugged with sebum.
13. An agent that inhibits the growth of microorganisms.
14. Oil in the skin.
15. To relieve itching.
16. To soften hardened skin and promote peeling and shedding.
17. To form a film over the skin.
18. a 19. f 20. b 21. e 22. h
23. d 24. g 25. c 26. i
27. Eczema (dermatitis)
28. Psoriasis
29. Seborrheic dermatitis
30. Decubitus
31. Pediculosis
32–33. Answers will vary depending on the edition of the *PDR*® used.

Chapter 8 Test Answers

1. d	2. c	3. a	4. d	5. b	6. c	7. d
8. b	9. d	10. a	11. d	12. d	13. a	14. c
15. c	16. a	17. c	18. b	19. a	20. d	21. d
22. b	23. c	24. e	25. a			

CHAPTER 9

Drugs for the Cardiovascular System

Objectives

- Name the parts of the cardiovascular system and state their functions.
- State the names of instruments used to measure blood pressure and to record the heartbeat.
- State the average blood pressure and pulse rate.
- List the main components of blood.
- State the functions of the lymphatic system.
- Identify the proper medical terms for common symptoms of cardiovascular disorders.
- Explain the major disorders for which cardiovascular drugs are given.
- Describe the actions and give examples of the following drug groups: vasopressors, vasodilators, diuretics, antihypertensives, calcium channel blockers, antilipemics, cardiac glycosides, antidysrhythmics, anticoagulants, thrombolytics, hemostatics, and hematinics.
- State the difference between an initial dose and a maintenance dose.
- Follow the proper procedure for administering oral and sublingual medications to patients with cardiovascular disorders.
- State the special procedures for administering adrenergics (vasoconstrictors), vasodilators, antihypertensives, digitalis, antidysrhythmics, anticoagulants, hemostatics, and hematinics.

Chapter Outline

Key Terms
Cardiovascular System
Cardiovascular Disorders
Drugs for Cardiovascular and Blood Disorders
Giving Cardiovascular Medications
Health Care for Today and Tomorrow
Legal and Ethical Care
Chapter 9 Review

Teaching Strategies

- Discuss the definitions of the key terms, making certain students are clear about their meaning.
- Have students work in cooperative learning groups to practice taking each other's pulse and blood pressure. Have them check each other for accuracy. Report abnormal readings.
- Show a film about the cardiovascular system.
- In the lab, display posters, charts, and other visuals of the heart and vascular system. Have students review them and name the classifications of car-

diovascular drugs that affect the parts of the cardiovascular system. Using visuals, ask students to show where certain disorders appear most often and what drugs are administered. Refer to the Representative Drugs table in the text.

- Set up an area in the lab for students to practice doing EKGs on each other. Ask them to compare their EKGs with one found in a reference text.
- Make arrangements for students to visit the EKG department of a hospital. Have them write a summary of what they learned. Discuss the drugs often used after an EKG.
- Ask the American Heart Association to send a speaker into class to discuss the proper care of the heart (smoking, diet, etc.). Ask the speaker to bring visuals for the presentation. Ask students to summarize the presentation in writing.
- Ask a nurse or physician from a Coronary Care Unit to talk with the students about the most commonly used cardiovascular drugs. Discuss how students will play an important role in the administration of these drugs or in helping other professionals administer them (pulse, BP, charting, elderly patients, etc.).
- In the lab, provide drug forms of various cardiovascular medications. Using the *PDR*® or other references, provide the manufacturer's label and picture for the following: *Catapress* patches; *Lanoxin* tabs; *Lanoxicaps; Sorbitrate* sublingual tabs; *Cardizem* tabs; *Isoptin IV;* and *Mevacor* tabs. Have students demonstrate administering them according to the following:

Want:	Have:	Give:
Catapress patch 0.6 mg	0.1 mg, 0.2 mg	(3) 0.2 mg
Lanoxin tabs 250 micro	125 micro	2 tabs
Lanoxicaps 600 micro	200 micro	3 caps
Sorbitrate subl 2.5 mg	2.5 mg	1 subl tab
Cardizem tabs 120 mg	30 mg	4 tabs
Isoptin IV 10 mg	2.5 ml/ampules	4 vials
Mevacor tab 50 mg	(10) 20-mg tabs	2.5 tabs

- Have students demonstrate Practice Procedure 9-1. Develop a checklist from the Practice Procedure to use in your assessment.
- Using charts, show the lymphatic system and compare its function to the cardiovascular system's function (location, filtering).
- Ask students to make posters (individually) showing the most common symptoms present in cardiovascular disease. Using the Representative Drugs table in the text, ask students to name the drugs most often administered for each disease.
- Arrange a trip to the emergency room of a hospital for a day. Have students record the patients they observe and the medications the patients are given. Ask them to write a summary of their observations including dose, actions, adverse effects, and special implications.
- Ask students to complete the Chapter 9 Review. Discuss answers and correct any misconceptions students may have. Review any material students had difficulty with.

- Administer and grade the Chapter 9 Test in this Instructor's Manual.
- Develop and administer a performance test on administering oral, sublingual, and buccal medications.

Critical Thinking Activities

1. You are caring for a patient who is being started on sublingual nitroglycerin tablets. The client experiences chest pain whenever he is under stress. What is the most likely cause of the angina? What instructions should you give the patient?
2. A patient in the hospital has just started taking an anticoagulant drug. What are your primary responsibilities to the client who is taking an anticoagulant?

Answers to Chapter 9 Review

1. Abnormal accumulation of fluids in the interstitial tissues.
2. Rapid heartbeat (over 100 beats per minute).
3. Slow heartbeat (fewer than 60 beats per minute).
4. High blood pressure, two or more systolic readings above 140 mm Hg.
5. Low blood pressure, systolic reading falls to 90 mm Hg or below.

6. b 7. a 8. e 9. d 10. c

11. point of maximum impulse
12. capillaries
13. deoxygenated
14. oxygenated
15. Shock
16. Atherosclerosis
17. Arteriosclerosis
18. Thrombophlebitis
19. Embolism
20. Angina pectoris
21. Myocardial infarction
22. tighten the blood vessel walls and raise blood pressure.
23. relax the blood vessel walls, dilate the arteries and veins.
24. strengthen the myocardium, increase force of contraction, slow the heart, improve muscle tone of myocardium.
25. stabilize heart muscle so it does not beat too rapidly.
26. prevent the blood clotting process.
27. promote blood clotting.
28. replace iron needed for red blood cell production.

29. a 30. b

31. bleeding, hemorrhage
32. Nitroglycerin
33. 60 per minute
34. faint, dizzy
35. stain

36–37. Answers will vary depending on the edition of the *PDR*® used and the specific drugs selected.

Chapter 9 Test Answers

1. F	2. F	3. T	4. T	5. F	6. T	7. b
8. a	9. f	10. d	11. e	12. c	13. d	14. c
15. a	16. b	17. a	18. b	19. d	20. a	21. b
22. a	23. c	24. c	25. d	26. d	27. a	28. a
29. d	30. b	31. d	32. d	33. a	34. d	35. b
36. c	37. d	38. b	39. b	40. d		

CHAPTER 10

Drugs for the Respiratory System

Objectives

- Name and describe the parts of the respiratory system.
- Give the normal respiration rate for an adult.
- Explain why coughing is important for maintaining a patient's airway.
- List and describe common symptoms of respiratory disorders, using correct medical terms.
- Recognize descriptions of the major respiratory disorders.
- Describe the actions and give examples of the following drug groups: antitussives, expectorants, decongestants, antihistamines, and bronchodilators.
- Define the three chest physiotherapy procedures.
- Administer nose drops using the correct procedure.
- Correctly administer oxygen therapy as ordered.

Chapter Outline

Key Terms
Respiratory System
Respiratory System Disorders
Drugs for Respiratory Disorders
Giving Respiratory Drugs
Health Care for Today and Tomorrow
Legal and Ethical Issues
Chapter 10 Review

Teaching Strategies

- Ask students to identify the key terms they are unfamiliar with. Discuss the definitions and be certain that students are clear about the meanings. Point out any similarities that may be confusing to students and tell them to memorize these words to avoid confusion later on.
- If possible, show films about the upper and lower respiratory systems. Discuss the physiology of the respiratory system and show its need for a normal functioning cardiovascular system to supply oxygen to the body.
- Demonstrate a noninvasive procedure for checking blood gas using an oximeter monitor on the ear, nose, and finger.
- Discuss medical implications for oxygen therapy that must be considered as the students administer medications to a patient on oxygen (i.e., checking for sores around mouth or nose, proper patient positioning after they administer drugs, maintaining appropriate rateflow, and checking for toxicity signs or restlessness).

- In the laboratory, have the students make a display of the heart/lung anatomy. Encourage them to work in cooperative learning groups. Have them memorize the way the blood travels from the lungs to the heart and back from the heart to the lungs and out into the body. They can make posters or use simulated lungs and heart that can be purchased.
- Invite a representative from the American Lung Association or state lung association to speak to the class. Ask the individual to bring pamphlets, slides, films, and/or lung models showing the damage done to the body by smoking. Have the students discuss in class what they have seen and how they can help in the smoking battle.
- Ask the respiratory therapy department of your clinical sites to allow individual students to visit to see the therapy given to patients in these units. Have students write a summary of the patients and the treatments observed. What rate of respirations were normal for each of the patients as related to the particular disorder?
- Using Table 10-1, have students make a list of OTC drugs commonly used for each category.
- Ask a heart and lung specialist to visit the class and talk about the most common respiratory diseases or disorders. Have the doctor show slides of different diseases and disorders and discuss the relationship of the environment to the disorders.
- Have students work in cooperative learning groups to design a "Stop Smoking" campaign for your school or clinic. Ask groups to share their plans. Encourage students to select one campaign and implement it.
- Have a speaker from the public health department visit and explain the rules and regulations that have not been followed in the past and what new regulations are being implemented now because of the increase in many of the old communicable diseases such as tuberculosis. What does the future hold for the health care workers in relation to care and drugs to be given for these diseases?
- Ask students to complete the Chapter 10 Review. Discuss answers, clearing up any misconceptions students may have. Review any material students had difficulty with.
- Administer and grade the Chapter 10 Test in this Instructor's Manual.

Critical Thinking Activities

1. You are teaching a mother how to give nose drops to a toddler. The mother is afraid to instill the drops and says it is mean to hold the toddler down to put the drops in. What should you do?
2. You have been assigned to teach a class to a group of high school students on the dangers of smoking. What should you teach?

Answers to Chapter 10 Review

1. Pertaining to the lungs.
2. Labored or difficult breathing.
3. Rapid breathing.
4. Stopped breathing.
5. Breathing too rapidly or deeply, hyperventilation.
6. Same as hyperpnea.
7. Membranes lining the lungs and lung cavities.
8. Symptoms returning in worse form after a drug has worn off.
9. respiration
10. pharynx
11. larynx
12. epiglottis
13. trachea
14. pronchi
15. alveoli
16. stethoscope
17. nebulizer or atomizer
18. Suppress coughing.

19. Liquify and reduce the viscosity of tenacious secretions.
20. Vasoconstrictors that shrink engorged nasal mucous membranes.

21. a	22. d	23. b	24. c	25. d
26. c	27. e	28. b	29. a	

30. The increase in HIV infection (HIV weakens the immune system), the development of drug resistant strains of tuberculosis, the immigration of people from countries where tuberculosis is prevalent, and the fact that many cases go untreated and are spread to others.
31. Expectorants keep sputum moist and thin. Bronchodilators promote coughing up sputum that may be clogging the air passages.

32. Tuberculosis	33. Asthma	34. Emphysema
35. Bronchitis	36. Pneumonia	

37–38. Answers will vary depending on the edition of the *PDR*® that is used.

Chapter 10 Test Answers

1. d	2. b	3. a	4. e	5. c	6. F	7. T
8. F	9. T	10. F	11. F	12. F	13. T	14. c
15. a	16. b	17. c	18. c	19. b	20. a	21. b
22. d	23. d	24. c	25. d	26. a	27. c	28. d
29. a	30. c	31. a	32. c			

CHAPTER 11

Drugs for the Gastrointestinal System

Objectives

- State the five main functions of the gastrointestinal system.
- Name the major parts of the gastrointestinal system and tell what they do.
- Use correct medical terms to describe symptoms of gastrointestinal disorders.
- Describe the major gastrointestinal disorders for which drugs are given.
- Discuss the actions and give examples of the following drug groups: antacids, histamine H_2-receptor antagonists, digestants, antiflatulents, emetics, antiemetics, anticholinergics and antispasmodics, antidiarrheals, laxatives, antihelmintics, and anorexiants.
- State three important conditions to be aware of when giving medications for the gastrointestinal system.
- Describe and follow proper procedure for inserting rectal suppositories.
- Describe and follow proper procedure for giving medications through a nasogastric or gastrostomy tube.

Chapter Outline

Key Terms
Gastrointestinal System
Disorders of the Gastrointestinal System
Drugs That Affect the Gastrointestinal System
Giving Gastrointestinal Medications
Health Care for Today and Tomorrow
Legal and Ethical Issues
Chapter 11 Review

Teaching Strategies

- Ask students to identify the key terms they are familiar with. Have volunteers use those terms in sentences. Discuss definitions of the unfamiliar terms and be certain that students are clear about the meanings. Point out any similarities that may be confusing.
- If possible, obtain and show a film, video, or slides of the gastrointestinal tract. Review the anatomy and physiology.
- If possible, obtain and show videos showing procedures for administering drugs via suppositories, colostomies, or a nasogastric and gastrostomy tube.
- Invite a nurse specializing in colostomy care to visit the class. Ask the nurse to discuss or bring a patient who can talk about his or her condition. Discuss drugs taken pre- and postoperatively. Ask students to summarize in writing the positive and negative benefits of a colostomy.
- Assign the students the project of listing the most common adverse effects of the OTC drugs listed in Table 11-1 in the text.
- Invite the nursing educator from the dietary department of one of your clinical sites to speak to the students about the most popular diets on the market now and the pros and cons of their effects.
- Arrange with a gastroenterologist's office for your students to individually observe the procedures performed in this office. Have the students summarize their visits and discuss the GI medications used most often for the most common disorders. Have students share their findings in class.
- Ask students to visit a health food store and bring back literature distributed there. How does it compare to medical information?
- Using Table 11-2 in the text, have each student choose a category that does not have a drug listed and list a drug from the Representative Drugs table that is in that category. If a drug is not listed, use the pharmacology resources to name some of them.
- In the laboratory provide drug forms of gastrointestinal drugs, and equipment needed to administer them. Use the *PDR*® picture section or any other resource. Try to get real gastrointestinal drug labels so you can put them on empty containers and ask the students to practice administering them. Ask for the following labels: *Dulcolax* 10 mg suppositories, *Tagamet* suspension 50 mg/ml, *Zantac* prefilled syringe of 2 ml/50 mg (25 mg/ml), *Tigan* 250 mg tab, *Cefobid* 2 g IV.
- Ask students to demonstrate administering the sample drugs using the following:

Have:	Want:	Give:
Dulcolax 10 mg supp.	20 mg	(2 supp)
Tagamet 50/mg susp.	150 mg PO	(3 ml)
Zantac 2 ml/50 mg IM prefilled syringe or 2 ml/50 mg IM vial or ampule	50 mg IM	(2 ml)
Zantac (as above)	25 mg IM	(1 ml)
Tigan 250 mg tab.	1 g PO	(4 tabs)
Cefobid 2 g vial IM/IV	1 g IM	(½ vial)

  Develop and administer a performance test for this activity.
- Ask students to complete the Chapter 11 Review. Discuss answers, clearing up any misconceptions students may have. Review any material students had difficulty with.
- Administer and grade the Chapter 11 Test in this Instructor's Manual.

Critical Thinking Activities

1. Simethicone (*Mylicon*) has been prescribed for a patient with flatulence. What else can you teach this patient to reduce flatulence? Give the rationale for your answer.
2. An elderly client has been taking sodium bicarbonate for indigestion and heartburn. Why is this of concern?

Answers to Chapter 11 Review

1. c   2. f   3. b   4. e   5. d   6. g   7. a
8. digestive
9. digestive tract, gastrointestinal tract, or alimentary canal
10. peristalsis
11. digestive juices, or enzymes
12. small intestine
13. saliva   14. esophagus
15. vomiting, or emesis   16. duodenum
17. villi   18. feces, or stools
19. anus   20. liver
21. gallbladder   22. pancreas
23. Breaking up food, transporting food through the system, secreting digestive enzymes, absorbing nutrients into the blood, and excreting solid wastes.
24. Enzyme secretion and peristalsis are controlled by the autonomic nervous system, which is also influenced by emotional stress.
25. Nausea, vomiting, indigestion, bloating, cramping, belching, flatus, constipation, abdominal pain, diarrhea, anorexia, weight loss, and changes in the appearance of stools.
26. Intestinal motility is the speed and force of peristalsis. Changes in motility lead to either diarrhea or constipation.
27. If eating and chewing are painful because of these problems, people will not eat correctly, and poor nutrition and constipation will result.
28. neutralize stomach acid.
29. supplement or replace digestive juices.
30. reduce gassiness and bloating.
31. stop vomiting and nausea.
32. slow peristalsis and block secretion of stomach acid.
33. relieve diarrhea by soaking up fluids or slowing peristalsis.
34. stimulate bowel movements or clear out the intestines.
35. destroy intestinal parasites (worms).
36. suppress the appetite.
37. f   38. b   39. e   40. a   41. h   42. d
43. g   44. c   45. i   46. j   47. k   48. l
49. Softening feces, stimulating peristalsis, adding bulk to the diet, and coating or lubricating.
50. Bland diet; 1500–2000 cc fluids daily; getting enough exercise; reducing nervous tension; giving up smoking, coffee, and alcohol.
51. Give medications at the proper time (before, after, or with meals or at bedtime). Give the right amount of liquid with each. Be wary of giving PRN medications for abdominal pain.

52. Provide privacy, explain what you are going to do, lubricate the suppository, and insert it gently and smoothly.
53. Signs of pain or infection, appearance of stools, and bowel movement too soon after insertion.
54. Crush tablets between two spoons or in a mortar and pestle and then mix with 1 oz of water. Open capsules and dissolve in water. Do not crush and dissolve timed-release tablets or capsules.
55. Signs of inflammation or leakage around the stoma or poor tube drainage.
56. Promotes defecation.
57. *Maalox, Mylanta, Gelusil*
58. Hemorrhoids
59. Hepatitis
60. Gallstones
61. Cirrhosis
62. Gastritis
63. Duodenal ulcer
64. Peritonitis
65. Irritable bowel

66–69. Answers will vary depending on the edition of the *PDR*® used.

Chapter 11 Test Answers

1. d	2. b	3. d	4. c	5. a	6. a	7. d
8. b	9. a	10. c	11. d	12. a	13. b	14. d
15. a	16. c	17. d	18. b	19. a	20. a	21. c
22. a	23. d	24. a	25. c	26. c	27. c	28. a
29. d						

CHAPTER 12

Drugs for the Urinary System and Fluid Balance

Objectives

- State three functions of the urinary system.
- Name the parts of the urinary system and tell what they do.
- Describe how abnormal alteration in the urine gives an indication to disorders in the urinary system.
- Give the correct medical terms for symptoms of urinary system disorders and fluid imbalances.
- Identify descriptions of the main disorders that affect the urinary system.
- Describe the actions and give examples of the following drug groups: urinary antiseptics, diuretics, and replacement electrolytes and fluids.
- Describe the patient care and education that goes with giving diuretics.
- State the purposes of a urinary catheter.
- Describe the causes of dehydration and the treatment in the pediatric patient.
- Follow proper procedure for administering medications through an indwelling catheter.

Chapter Outline

Key Terms
Urinary System
Disorders of the Kidneys and the Urinary Tract

Imbalances of Body Fluids, Electrolytes, and pH
Drugs for the Urinary Tract and Fluid Imbalances
Giving Drugs That Affect the Urinary System
Health Care for Today and Tomorrow
Legal and Ethical Issues
Chapter 12 Review

Teaching Strategies

- Ask students to define the key terms. Discuss the definitions, and be certain that students are clear about the meanings.
- Show a film or video of the urinary system. Discuss the physiology and the disorders of the urinary system.
- Have students work in cooperative learning groups in the laboratory to practice administering medications through a urinary catheter.
- Develop and administer a performance test for administering medications through a urinary catheter.
- Ask students to make a visual display of the urinary system. Have them work in small groups to memorize the functions of the Loop of Henle as it relates to proper fluid balance of the body.
- In the laboratory, provide the drug forms of the urinary drugs as well as the equipment needed to administer them. Use the *PDR*® or other resources for pictures or labels that can be put on the containers, or ask a pharmacist to supply labels. Ask for *Bactrim DS; HydroDIURIL* 25 mg tabs; *Lasix* 40 mg/4 ml vial, ampule, or prefilled syringe; Furosemide 40 mg/4 ml vial, ampule, or prefilled syringe; *Lasix* susp, 10 mg/ml; Hydrochlorothiazide 25 mg and 50 mg tabs; *Macrodantin* 100 mg tabs. Have students demonstrate administering the sample drugs using the following:

Have:	Want:	Give:
Bactrim DS/Regular	*Bactrim* DS PO	(1 DS or 2 reg tabs)
HydroDIURIL 25 mg tabs	*HydroDIURIL* 100 mg PO	(4 tabs)
Lasix 40 mg/4 ml/IM	*Lasix* 40 mg IM	(1 4-ml amp or 4 ml from vial or prefilled syringe)
Furosemide 10 mg/ml/IV	Furosemide 10 mg IV	(1-ml amp, vial or prefilled syringe)
Furosemide 10 mg/ml/IM	Furosemide .01 g IM	(1-ml amp, vial or prefilled syringe)
Lasix 15/ml mg susp.	15 mg/ml susp.	(1 ml)
Hydrochlorothiazide 25–50 mg tabs	0.1 g PO	(2 50-mg tabs)
Macrodantin 100 mg tabs.	0.1 g PO	(1 100-mg tab)

- Using the Representative Drugs table in the book, discuss the condition of CHF and the relationship of diuretics.
- Ask the students to complete the Chapter 12 Review. Discuss answers, clearing up any misconceptions students may have. Review any material students had difficulty with.
- Administer and grade the Chapter 12 Test in this Instructor's Manual.

Critical Thinking Activities

1. What are two potential problems that may occur with diuretic therapy? What can you do to prevent these problems?
2. Discuss why small children are more susceptible to the effects of diuretics and fluid and electrolyte imbalances.
3. A 10-month-old infant has a fever, vomiting, and three times as many stools as usual. The stools are watery in consistency. The child is evaluated to be dehydrated because of acute infectious diarrhea. What is the recommended treatment in this situation?

Answers to Chapter 12 Review

1. Blood in the urine.
2. Pus in the urine.
3. Inability to control urination.
4. Inability to urinate even when the bladder is full.
5. Painful urination.
6. No production of urine.

7. b 8. a 9. d 10. c

11. ureters 12. urethra 13. urinate, or void

14. 1500–2000 15. 250 16. potassium

17. bananas or oranges
18. indwelling, anchored, or retention
19. Excreting waste products of metabolism (urea, mineral salts), regulating the amount of water in the body, and regulating the pH.
20. Electrolytes are ions of mineral salts that provide the chemical transport system for cell metabolism. Examples: calcium, sodium, potassium, magnesium, chloride, bicarbonate, phosphate, and sulfate.
21. By controlling the reabsorption process so that excess electrolytes and fluids are excreted in the urine.
22. Input: water, juice, IV fluids, gastrostomy fluids
    Output: urine, vomitus, wound drainage, stomach suction, diarrhea

23. e 24. g 25. c 26. d 27. h 28. a 29. b 30. f

31. Renal failure 32. Kidney stones 33. Cystitis

34. Pyelonephritis 35. Electrolyte imbalance

36–37. Answers will vary depending on the edition of the *PDR*® used.

Chapter 12 Test Answers

1. b	2. c	3. a	4. c	5. d	6. d	7. b
8. d	9. d	10. b	11. c	12. a	13. d	14. d
15. d	16. c	17. d	18. b	19. d	20. b	21. a
22. d	23. a	24. d	25. b	26. c	27. d	

CHAPTER 13

Drugs for the Reproductive System

Objectives

- Name the main parts of the male and female internal and external genitalia.
- Identify the parts and functions of the reproductive system, using correct medical terminology.
- Discuss the effects of puberty on the adolescent patient and the need for contraceptive counseling.
- Name the hormones produced by the male and female gonads and describe their function.
- Describe the actions of gonadotropins, oxytocin, and prolactin.
- Recognize descriptions of major disorders that affect the reproductive system.

- List the main uses of sex hormones in drug therapy.
- State the major side effects of hormone therapy.

Chapter Outline

Key Terms
Reproductive System
Disorders of the Reproductive System
Use of Sex Hormone in Drug Therapy
Health Care for Today and Tomorrow
Legal and Ethical Issues
Chapter 13 Review

Teaching Strategies

- Ask students to identify key terms they are unfamiliar with. Discuss the definitions and be certain that students are clear about the meanings.
- Show a film on the reproductive system. Discuss the physiology of the system. If possible, show a film that demonstrates administering medications vaginally. Have the students work in small groups in the laboratory practicing administering medications vaginally. Develop and administer a test for administering medications vaginally.
- Ask the students to make a display of the reproductive system. Let them work in small groups to memorize the hormones that regulate reproduction.
- In the laboratory, provide the reproductive drugs and the equipment needed to administer them. Use the *PDR*® or other resources for pictures or labels that can be put on the bottles and other containers. Use the following drugs and drug doses: *Femstat* 2 percent vaginal cream, *Monistat* 0.2 supp, *Estraderm* patch 0.05 mg, *Premarin* 2.5 mg tabs, *Flagyl* 250 mg tabs, *Demulen* 1/35, 21–28 tabs, *Provera* 5 mg tabs. Have students demonstrate administering the sample drugs using the following:

Have:	**Want:**	**Give:**
Femstat 5 g of 2% vag. cr.	5 g	(1 applicator)
Monistat 0.2 supp	0.2 g	(1 supp)
Estraderm 0.05 mg/patch	0.10 mg	(2 patches)
Premarin 2.5 mg tabs	10 mg	(4 tabs)
Flagyl 500 mg tabs	1 g	(2 tabs)
Demulen 1/35, 21–28	1/35	(1 tab)
Provera 5 mg tabs	2.5 mg	($\frac{1}{2}$ tab)

- Use the Representative Drugs table in the text to discuss the present theory on prescribing hormones for menopause because of surgery or because of natural menopause.
- Ask the students to complete the Chapter 13 Review. Discuss answers, clearing up any misconceptions students may have. Review any material students had difficulty with.
- Administer and grade the Chapter 13 Test in this Instructor's Manual.

Critical Thinking Activities

1. Why are oxytocics such as *Pitocin* used in the postpartum period?
2. Discuss ways of obtaining educational materials for both schools and communities on sexually transmitted diseases.

Answers to Chapter 13 Review

1. Drug that induces or strengthens labor.
2. Painful menstruation.
3. Swelling of breasts with milk or swelling of the penis prior to ejaculation.
4. Lining of the uterus.
5. Anything used to terminate pregnancy.

6. Human immunodeficiency virus.
7. Acquired immune deficiency syndrome.

8. ovaries	9. testes	10. vagina	11. uterus
12. mammary	13. prostate	14. urethra	
15. d	16. b	17. a	18. c

19. Easing menopause symptoms, osteoporosis, amenorrhea, prevention of breast engorgement, senile vaginitis, uterine bleeding, endometriosis, contraception, breast and prostate cancer, hormone replacement, reversal of tissue wasting.
20. Nausea, breakthrough bleeding, water retention, vaginal infections, headache, risk of blood clots, possible cancer link, feminization of males.
21. Masculinization of females, water retention.

22. F	23. F	24. T	25. T	26. F	27. T	28. T	29. T

30. Cervicitis
31. Benign prostatic hypertrophy (BPH)
32. Endometriosis
33. Acquired immune deficiency syndrome (AIDS)
34. Genital herpes simplex

35–36. Answers will vary depending on the edition of the *PDR*® that is used.

Chapter 13 Test Answers

1. a	2. b	3. b	4. a	5. a	6. a	7. b
8. c	9. a	10. d	11. b	12. d	13. b	14. c
15. c	16. a	17. a	18. d	19. a	20. d	21. b
22. d	23. a	24. c	25. d			

CHAPTER 14

Drugs for the Endocrine System

Objectives

- Name the hormones produced by the seven major glands.
- State the action of each of these hormones or hormonelike drugs: somatotropic hormone, thyroxine, parathyroid, corticosteroids, epinephrine (adrenaline) and norepinephrine, insulin, adrenocorticotropic hormone, and antidiuretic hormone.
- State which hormones are lacking in the condition of diabetes mellitus, diabetes insipidus, Addison's disease, and hypothyroidism, and give examples of drugs used for replacement in each case.
- Use correct medical terms in referring to parts of the endocrine system and symptoms of hormone imbalances.
- List the types of insulin available for treatment of diabetes mellitus, and give examples of each group.
- Give examples of oral hypoglycemics used for diabetes treatment and explain how they work.

- Recognize the symptoms of hyperglycemia and hypoglycemia and explain how they are treated.
- State what factors affect the insulin needs of a patient with diabetes mellitus.
- List at least three uses of corticosteroids.
- Name five possible side effects of long-term corticosteroid therapy.

Chapter Outline

Key Terms
Endocrine System
Disorders of the Endocrine System
Hormone Therapy
Administering Insulin
Health Care for Today and Tomorrow
Legal and Ethical Issues
Chapter 14 Review

Teaching Strategies

- Ask students to demonstrate their knowledge of key terms.
- Discuss the physiology of the endocrine system and the common disorders.
- Show a film on administering insulin. Discuss the procedures, then let the students practice administering insulin in small groups. Develop and administer a performance test.
- Have the students prepare a list of drugs that commonly interact with insulin.
- Ask a representative from the American Diabetes Association to visit the class and discuss the various aspects of diabetes and its management. Have the representative distribute brochures to the students.
- Using the Representative Drugs table in the text, ask the students to identify the different drugs given for diabetes insipidus and diabetes mellitus.
- In the laboratory, provide the drugs and equipment needed to administer them. Use the *PDR*® or other resources for pictures or labels that can be put on the containers. Use drugs as follows: *Glucotrol* 10 mg tabs, *Deltasone* 2.5 mg and 5 mg tabs, *K-Lor* 20 mEq packs, *Regular* insulin 100 units vial, *Lente* insulin 100 units vial, *Calcimar* 200 IU/ml vial, *Synthroid* 200 mcg IV and diluent, *Levothroid* 25 mcg tabs. Develop and administer a performance test for administering the following:

Have:	Want:	Give:
Glucotrol 10 mg tabs.	2 mg	(2 tabs)
Deltasone 2.5 mg tabs.	5 mg	(2 tabs)
K-Lor 20 mEq	60 mEq	(3 tabs)
Regular insulin 100 U/vial	50 units	(Use insulin syringe and give 0.5 ml)
Lente insulin 100 U/ml per ml	22 units	(Use insulin syringe and give 22 units)
Regular and *Lente* insulin 100 U vial each	5 U Reg. 25 U *Lente*	(See insulin and mix wanted dose—R first then add L)
Calcimar 200 IU/ml	100 IU/SQ	(0.5 ml SQ)
Synthroid 200 mcg	200 mcg	(See *PDR*® for diluent and amount)
Levothroid 25 mcg tabs	75 mcg	(3 tabs)

- Ask students to complete the Chapter 14 Review. Discuss answers, clearing up any misconceptions students may have. Review any material students had difficulty with.
- Administer and grade the Chapter 14 Test in this Instructor's Manual.

Critical Thinking Activities

1. A 200-pound, 35-year-old woman has just been diagnosed with Type I diabetes mellitus. The physician placed her on a 1500-calorie diabetic diet and 30 units of NPH insulin at 7:30 A.M. every day. At 4:00 P.M., the patient states she is weak and sweaty. How would you explain these symptoms to the patient?
2. Discuss the similarities and differences in caring for Type I diabetes mellitus and Type II diabetes mellitus.

Answers to Chapter 14 Review

1. Muscle spasms or twitching.
2. Sugar in the urine.
3. Low blood sugar.
4. Hormone secreted by the beta cells in the islets of Langerhans in the pancreas; regulates the use of sugar by body cells.
5. Hormone secreted by the pancreas that raises the level of blood sugar; counteracts the effects of insulin.
6. Form of sugar stored in the liver or muscles for release as the body needs it.

7. c 8. e 9. d 10. a 11. b

12. thyroid 13. adrenal 14. insulin 15. antidiuretic

16. adrenal, or corticosteroid

17. L 18. I 19. O 20. F 21. I 22. O 23. F 24. F

25. Oral hypoglycemics stimulate the pancreas to produce more insulin.
26. The main factors are diet, exercise, and emotions. Infection, ketoacidosis, and other disorders are also factors.
27. Glucocorticoids regulate the use of fat and sugar by the body, and mineralocorticoids regulate the salt/water balancing function of the kidneys.
28. Hormone replacement, suppression of immune response, inflammation and allergic reaction, skin inflammations, eye and respiratory diseases.
29. Delayed wound healing, peptic ulcer, rounded (moon) face, euphoria, weight gain, insomnia, edema, muscle weakness, hypokalemia.

30. a 31. c 32. b

33. Problem: Elevated blood glucose. Give insulin.
34. Problem: Low blood glucose. Give sugar (orange juice, soft drink, candy, etc.).

35–36. Answers will vary depending on the edition of the *PDR*® used.

Chapter 14 Test Answers

1. b	2. a	3. a	4. b	5. c	6. b	7. a
8. a	9. c	10. c	11. d	12. b	13. d	14. a
15. b	16. d	17. a	18. d	19. a	20. b	21. d
22. d	23. d	24. a	25. c	26. d	27. c	28. b
29. a	30. b					

CHAPTER 15

Drugs for the Musculoskeletal System

Objectives

- Use correct medical terms to describe major parts, functions, and disorders of the musculoskeletal system.
- Recognize descriptions of major disorders that affect the musculoskeletal system.
- Explain the differences among gout, osteoarthritis, and rheumatoid arthritis.
- Describe the actions of drug groups commonly used in the treatment of gout, osteoarthritis, and rheumatoid arthritis, and give examples.
- Identify the side effects of the various drug categories used to treat musculoskeletal disorders.
- Describe malfunctions of bone marrow and their effects on blood.
- Describe the usual nursing care of patients with musculoskeletal disorders.

Chapter Outline

Key Terms
Musculoskeletal System
Drug Treatment of Musculoskeletal Disorders
Care of Patients with Musculoskeletal Disorders
Health Care for Today and Tomorrow
Legal and Ethical Issues
Chapter 15 Review

Teaching Strategies

- Ask students to define each of the key terms. Discuss the definitions and be certain that students are clear about the meanings.
- Discuss the physiology of the musculoskeletal system.
- Show a film on disorders of the musculoskeletal system.
- In the laboratory, provide the drugs and equipment to administer drugs for the musculoskeletal system. Use the *PDR*® or other resources for pictures and labels that can be put on the containers. Use the Representative Drugs table in the text for the following drugs and doses to practice giving in the laboratory: Aspirin 325 mg tab, Ibuprofen 25 mg tab, Indomethacin 25 mg tabs, *Naproxen* 500 mg tabs, Aspirin 325 mg supp. Have students demonstrate administration of the following:

Have:	Want:	Give:
Aspirin 325 mg tabs	Aspirin 325 g	(1 tab)
Ibuprofen 25 mg tabs	Ibuprofen 100 mg	(4 tabs)
Indomethacin 25 mg tabs	Indomethacin 50 mg	(2 tabs)
Naproxen 500 mg tabs	*Naproxen* 750 mg	($1\frac{1}{2}$ tabs)
Aspirin 325 mg supp	Aspirin 325 mg supp	(1 supp)

- Ask students to complete the Chapter 15 Review. Discuss answers, clearing up any misconceptions students may have. Review any material students had difficulty with.
- Administer and grade the Chapter 15 Test in this Instructor's Manual.

Critical Thinking Activities

1. You are caring for a postmenopausal woman. Develop a plan to educate the patient on the prevention of osteoporosis.
2. Develop a daily menu for a patient with gout.

Answers to Chapter 15 Review

1. Drug that reduces the formation of uric acid.
2. A drug that controls muscle spasms.
3. Wasting and decrease in size of muscle (e.g., atrophy of a muscle due to lack of use).
4. An injury that can occur when muscles or tendons are subjected to stress, especially if stress lasts for a period of time.
5. An injury that can result from violent stress on a ligament.
6. Small, fluid-filled sacs that cushion spots where bones and muscles rub together.

7. move	8. ligaments	9. calcium
10. tendons	11. marrow	12. protect, support
13. skeletal	14. tone	15. sprains

16. d	17. a	18. c	19. b	20. F	21. T	22. T
23. F	24. F	25. T	26. T	27. F	28. T	29. T

30. Give pain medications on time, move patients carefully, don't bump the bed, meet their psychological needs.

31. Osteoporosis 32. Osteomyelitis 33. Bursitis 34. Gout

35–36. Answers will vary depending on the edition of the *PDR*® used.

Chapter 15 Test Answers

1. a	2. c	3. a	4. b	5. d	6. a	7. a
8. b	9. a	10. d	11. d	12. a	13. a	14. d
15. c	16. a	17. d	18. c	19. b	20. d	21. a
22. c						

CHAPTER 16

Drugs for the Nervous and Sensory Systems

Objectives

- Name the two main divisions of the nervous system and their parts.
- State the basic functions of the autonomic nervous system.
- Give the correct medical terms for symptoms of nervous system disorders.
- Recognize descriptions of the major nervous system disorders for which medications are given.
- Teach patients about preventing strokes.
- Teach the patient about the effects of caffeine.
- Describe the actions and give examples of the following drug groups: central nervous system stimulants, analgesics, anticonvulsants, and antiparkinsonian drugs.
- Follow general instructions for administering pain medications, long-term medications, stimulants, and emergency drugs.

Chapter Outline

Key Terms
The Nervous and Sensory Systems
Nervous System Disorders
Drugs That Affect the CNS
Giving Medications for the Nervous and Sensory Systems
Health Care for Today and Tomorrow
Legal and Ethical Issues
Chapter 16 Review

Teaching Strategies

- Ask students to identify the key terms they are familiar with. Discuss all of the definitions and be certain that students are clear about meanings. Point out any similarities that may be confusing to students.
- Have students get in groups and explore their feelings and attitudes toward the use of analgesics and their potential for abuse.
- In the laboratory, provide drug forms of respiratory medications. Using the *PDR®* or any other source, provide the original manufacturer's label or pictures for the following medications and have the student demonstrate administering these.

Physician wants:	You have:	You give:
Phenergan Rectal Suppositories 25 mg	12.5 mg suppositories	(2 supp)
Phenergan 100 mg PO	25 mg tabs	(4 tab)
Tylenol with Codeine Elix. 1 T	120 mg *Tylenol*/ 12 mg codeine/5ml (1 pint total)	(15 ml)
Morphine Sulfate SR 15 mg	30 mg tabs	($\frac{1}{2}$ ml)
Roxanol Oral Solution 25 mg	100 mg/4 ml	(1 ml)
Dilaudid-HP 25 mg Subcutaneous	50 mg/5 ml	($2\frac{1}{2}$ ml)

Develop and administer a performance test for this project.

- Request a flow sheet for patient-controlled analgesia from your clinical sites. Discuss how this is filled out.
- Ask students to complete the Chapter 16 Review. Discuss answers, clearing up any misconceptions students may have. Review any material students had difficulty with.
- Administer and grade the Chapter 16 Test in this Instructor's Manual.

Critical Thinking Activities

1. You are caring for a patient in the terminal stages of breast cancer. Discuss the role of a patient-controlled analgesic (PCA) pump in this patient's pain management.
2. Develop a teaching plan to be used with patients on the prevention of strokes.

Answers to Chapter 16 Review

1. Shakiness, trembling.
2. Dizziness.
3. Inability to move.
4. Deep sleep out of which a person cannot be roused.
5. Dazed condition, mental sluggishness.
6. Sleeplessness.
7. Slowness of movement.
8. Uncontrolled large muscle movement.
9. central, peripheral

10. spinal cord
11. autonomic
12. impulses or messages
13. relieve pain.
14. reduce fever.
15. control or prevent seizures.
16. c 17. d 18. a 19. b 20. e
21. take their medication regularly
22. toxicity or poisoning
23. on time
24. discard
25. temperature
26. candy or sugarless gum
27. Parkinson's disease
28. Multiple sclerosis (MS)
29. Stroke or CVA
30. Epilepsy
31. Meningitis

32–33. Answers will vary depending on the edition of the *PDR*® used.

Chapter 16 Test Answers

1. b	2. d	3. d	4. a	5. d	6. b	7. c
8. b	9. c	10. a	11. d	12. d	13. c	14. d
15. b	16. c	17. d	18. b	19. d		

CHAPTER 17 Psychotropic Drugs

Objectives

- Describe the biochemical mechanisms of the central nervous system that affect emotions.
- Define the correct medical terms for symptoms of mental disorders.
- Recognize descriptions of the major mental disorders.
- Differentiate between when a sedative is recommended and when a hypnotic is recommended.
- Describe the actions and give examples of the following drug groups: antidepressants, sedatives/hypnotics, antipsychotics, antianxiety drugs, and antimanics.
- Teach the patient about the appropriate administration of lithium.
- Follow general instructions for administering sedatives/hypnotics, antidepressants, antianxiety drugs, antipsychotics, and antimanics.
- Identify drugs that are often involved in drug abuse.

Chapter Outline

Key Terms
The Nervous System and Emotions
Mental Disorders
Selection and Use of Psychotropic Drugs
Giving Medications
Health Care for Today and Tomorrow
Legal and Ethical Issues
Chapter 17 Review

Teaching Strategies

- Arrange students into four cooperative learning groups. Have a different group discuss why a patient would receive an antipsychotic, antianxiety, antidepressant, or antimanic drug.

- Have each group develop a table on the use, usual dose, contraindications, and side effects of their drug. Bring the groups back together and have each group discuss their assigned drug.
- Show the video *One Flew Over the Cuckoo's Nest.* Point out that portrayals of patients in psychiatric settings are often uncomfortable. After the film, have students discuss the feelings the film evoked.
- Ask students to discuss the myths and stigmas about psychiatric patients and their treatment. Discuss how they can dispel these misconceptions.
- Ask students to explore how they would feel if they were told they needed to take a psychiatric drug.
- Ask a psychologist to visit the class and discuss both pharmacological and nonpharmacological methods of treating depression, manic-depression, and schizophrenia.
- Administer and grade the Chapter 17 Test in this Instructor's Manual.

Critical Thinking Activities

1. Discuss why it is necessary to obtain a nutritional history before administering a monamine oxidase (MAO) inhibitor to a patient.
2. Develop a plan to eliminate the extrapyramidal side effects that may occur with antipsychotic drugs.
3. Develop a teaching plan for a patient taking Lithium.

Answers to Chapter 17 Review

1. d 2. c 3. b 4. a
5. A state of feeling apprehensive, uneasy, uncertain, or a fear of the unknown.
6. Disorder characterized by a sense of worthlessness or hopelessness.
7. Mood disorder characterized by grandiose behavior, flight of ideas, poor judgment, and aggressiveness.
8. Disorder in which psychosis is a classic feature.
9. acetylcholine, norepinephrine
10. Neurohormones
11. inhibitory, excitatory
12. used in treatment of bipolar disorders.
13. relieve depression.
14. produce sleep.
15. produce feelings of calm in tense or nervous (but not psychotic) patients.
16. control agitated, hyperactive, destructive mentally ill patients.
17. another term for antipsychotic.
18. b 19. a 20. f 21. d 22. e 23. c
24. extrapyramidal symptoms
25. alcohol
26. salt
27. Reduce the noise level. Give a warm bath or a back rub. Listen to the patient's concerns. Give the patient enough exercise.
28. See the section on Drug Abuse.
29. Alcohol, cheese, liver.
30. Anxiety
31. Psychosis
32. Depression

Chapter 17 Test Answers

33–34. Answers will vary depending on the edition of the *PDR*® used.

1. b	2. d	3. a	4. c	5. d	6. b	7. a
8. c	9. b	10. c	11. d	12. a	13. d	14. b
15. d	16. c	17. b	18. a	19. d	20. a	21. b

CHAPTER 18
Antineoplastic Drugs

Objectives

- Use proper terms for discussing cells, tissues, organs, and body systems.
- Name the four types of body cells.
- Name the three characteristics of all cancers.
- Explain how chemotherapy works.
- List common antineoplastic drugs and their effects on the cell cycle.
- List the side effects to look for when working with patients on chemotherapy.
- Name at least three groups of antineoplastic drugs and give examples.

Chapter Outline

Key Terms
Body Systems
Necessary Substances
Immunity
Cancer and Chemotherapy
Health Care for Today and Tomorrow
Legal and Ethical Issues
Chapter 18 Review

Teaching Strategies

- Discuss definitions of the key terms. Point out any similarities that may be confusing to students.
- Ask students to refer to the Representative Drugs table at the end of the chapter. Discuss ways in which this resource will be helpful. Ask students if they have any difficulty reading it. If so, take the time to answer their questions.
- Divide students into two groups. Have one group develop a chart outlining the characteristics of benign tumors. Have the other group develop a chart outlining the characteristics of cancerous tumors. Have a representative from each group present the differences.
- Discuss the health care worker's responsibility in helping to prevent extravasation by antineoplastics and why it seems to be more important with this type of drug classification.
- Ask students to list the major complications of antineoplastic drug therapy. Discuss the care for each.
- Ask students to list different methods of oral hygiene suitable for cancer patients. (Consider where the cancer is located.)
- Invite an individual who is on or has recently completed chemotherapy to speak to the class about his or her experiences including how health care workers were helpful and how they were not helpful. Ask students to write a summary of the presentation including their own reactions. Discuss how caring for a patient with cancer is different from caring for other patients.

- Have students write up a case study on a patient with cancer. Tell students to include all cancer drugs the patient is taking and reasons for the use of multiple drugs.
- Ask students to complete the Chapter 18 Review. Discuss answers, clearing up any misconceptions students may have. Review any material students had difficulty with.
- Administer and grade the Chapter 18 Test in this Instructor's Manual.

Critical Thinking Activities

1. You are caring for a chemotherapy patient. Develop a plan of care for this patient.
2. How can you help a patient psychologically who has been diagnosed with cancer?

Answers to Chapter 18 Review

1. Reduction in the number of leukocytes in the blood, 4000 or less.
2. Basic unit of structure of all living things.
3. Poisonous to cells.
4. Abnormal lump or mass of tissue.
5. Drug therapy for cancer symptoms.
6. Ability of malignant cells to spread to other parts of the body.
7. Cancerous.
8. Loss of hair.
9. A well-defined tumor that is contained and will not spread to other parts of the body.
10. Cancerous, able to spread to other parts of the body.

11. c 12. a 13. b 14. d 15. e 16. f

17. They grow and divide more rapidly than normal cells. They invade nearby healthy tissues. They metastasize (spread) to other parts of the body.
18. Parts of the body where cells are dividing rapidly, such as the blood-forming areas of the bones.

19. c 20. a 21. d 22. b

23. Gastrointestinal upset (nausea, vomiting, diarrhea), pain, fever, and infections.

24–32. Answers will vary depending on the edition of the *PDR*® that is used.

Chapter 18 Test Answers

1. a	2. b	3. a	4. b	5. d	6. d	7. c
8. b	9. c	10. c	11. a	12. d	13. b	14. c
15. d	16. a	17. c	18. a	19. b	20. c	21. a
22. d	23. d					

CHAPTER 19

Administering Parenteral Medications

Objectives

- Apply Standard Precautions.
- Name and describe the major routes of parenteral administration.
- Identify the parts of a needle and syringe.

- List the appropriate sizes of needles and syringes for different types and sites of injection.
- Accurately identify dosages in calibrated syringes.
- Dispose of injection equipment properly.
- Draw up medications from ampules and vials, using aseptic technique.
- Follow instructions for reconstituting and storing parenteral medications.
- Locate the most common injection sites for intradermal, subcutaneous, and intramuscular administration.
- Describe and follow proper procedures for carrying out intradermal, subcutaneous, and intramuscular injections.
- Explain what to do when blood is aspirated during an injection.

Chapter Outline

Key Terms
Orientation to the Parenteral Route
Standard Precautions
Equipment
Drawing Up Medications
Injection Sites
General Procedure for Injections
Special Instructions
Health Care for Today and Tomorrow
Legal and Ethical Issues
Chapter 19 Review

Teaching Strategies

- Ask students to identify the key terms they are unfamiliar with. Discuss the definitions and be certain that students are clear about meanings.
- Show any films or slides you may have of administering medications by the parenteral routes.
- Review Table 19-1 on Universal Blood and Body Fluid Precautions and discuss their importance in the practice of administering parenteral medications.
- Have students practice giving injections a number of times before they are tested on the performance of the tasks. (You will need standard hypodermic 3 cc/ml syringes with 3/8 to $1\frac{1}{2}$ inch, 22 to 25 gauge needles, insulin syringes, tuberculin syringes, Tubex syringes, and alcohol swabs.) Purchase sterile empty ampules and vials from a pharmaceutical company if you cannot buy them at a medical supply company. Label them as insulins, narcotics, and other medications, such as vitamins and antibiotics. Purchase puncture-resistant containers.
- Hang posters, charts, and different types of visual aids showing proper handwashing technique; intradermal, subcutaneous, and intramuscular routes; equipment and procedures.
- Develop and administer performance tests for giving intradermal, subcutaneous, and intramuscular injections.
- Ask students to complete the Chapter 19 Review. Discuss answers, clearing up any misconceptions students may have. Review any material students had difficulty with.
- Administer and grade the Chapter 19 Test in this Instructor's Manual.

Critical Thinking Activities

1. You are preparing to give a patient an injection. The patient is afraid. What can you do to help the patient?
2. Discuss what you would do differently when giving a subcutaneous injection to an obese patient.

Answers to Chapter 19 Review

1. Consistent application of procedures for contact with blood and body fluids of all patients.
2. To suction; to pull back on the syringe plunger to check for entry into a blood vessel.
3. Thick and sticky.
4. Thin and watery.
5. a. tip; b. barrel; c. flange; d. plunger; e. bevel; f. needle cover or sheath; g. shaft, stem, or cannula; h. hub
6. a. 21 minims; b. 0.25 cc; c. 1.7 cc; d. 32 U
7. a. standard hypodermic; b. tuberculin; c. standard hypodermic; d. insulin
8.

	Intradermal	Subcutaneous	Intramuscular
a.	skin, dermis	subcutaneous, fatty tissue	muscle
b.	tuberculin	standard hypodermic or insulin	standard hypodermic
c.	$\frac{3}{8}$-inch	$\frac{3}{8}$—$\frac{5}{8}$-inch	1–1$\frac{1}{2}$-inch
d.	25–26G	24–26G	aqu. 21–23G visc. 18–20 G
e.	15°	45° or 90°	90°

9. Because rapid absorption is desired; because the drug is destroyed by digestive juices if taken orally; because the patient is unable to swallow, is unconscious, or has nausea, vomiting, or intestinal obstruction.
10. To pull back on the plunger and check for blood in the syringe after the needle is inserted into tissue; done to see whether the needle has entered a blood vessel.
11. Never administer a syringe with blood. Dispose of the syringe and start over.
12. d
13. a
14. c
15. b
16. sciatic
17. up
18. air
19. broken off
20. time, date, strength
21. See text.
22. Redness, rash, lumpiness, sloughing, necrosis, abscess.
23. Do not give the injection, but chart the appearance of the skin and consult the nurse in charge.
24. Answers will vary.
25. Ceftazidime.
26. Aerobes, gram-negative and gram-positive, anaerobes.
27. Lower respiratory tract infection, skin and skin structure, urinary tract infections, bacterial septicemia, bone and joint infection, gynecological infections, intra-abdominal infections, and central nervous system infections.
28. When the patient is hypersensitive to ceftazidime.

Chapter 19 Test Answers

1. needle cover
2. bevel
3. gauge number
4. tip
5. barrel
6. plunger
7. flange
8. plunger end

9. d	10. c	11. d	12. d	13. b	14. d	15. c
16. a	17. b	18. c	19. d	20. a	21. b	22. a
23. a	24. c	25. d	26. b	27. a	28. d	29. b
30. d	31. b	32. c	33. c	34. c	35. d	

CHAPTER 20

Drugs for the Geriatric Patient

Objectives

- Describe the major changes that take place in the various body systems during aging.
- State why treatment of elderly patients must be individualized according to each person's needs.
- Describe the effects of aging on absorption, distribution, metabolism, and excretion of drugs.
- Explain how medication orders are usually adjusted to account for the pharmacokinetics of an older patient.
- Explain why the presence of more diseases in old age makes drug therapy more complicated.
- State what types of adverse reactions health care workers must look for in administering drugs to the aged.
- Explain how elderly patients are affected by the attitudes and actions of health care workers.
- Review safe medication administration practices and the principles that are specific for the elderly patient.
- List ways that patients can take an active part in their own medication therapy.

Chapter Outline

Key Terms
Drugs and the Elderly
The Aging Process
Pharmacokinetics in the Aged
Administering Medications to Elderly Patients
Engaging Patients in Their Care
Health Care for Today and Tomorrow
Legal and Ethical Issues
Chapter 20 Review

Teaching Strategies

- Ask students to define the key terms they are unfamiliar with. Discuss the definitions and be certain that students are clear about the meanings.
- Using Table 20-1 in the text, ask students for the common interactions of drug therapy they have seen in older family members or those patients they may already be caring for.
- Contact the Department of Education in your state and ask about the guidelines for health care workers administering medications in long-term care facilities. Ask specifically about Certified Medication Aide. Does the state

have a written Medication Aide Course with a required number of hours of administering medications under supervision? Have health care workers taken a course in Nurse Aide training? (This is important because they must learn to take vital signs to be able to administer some drugs, such as *Lanoxin.*)

- Invite a director of nurses from a long-term care facility who is involved with the supervision of medication aide students to visit the class. Have him or her explain the importance of this new allied health worker. Be sure the director is supportive of this team member and is working with the state to upgrade the care in the long-term care facility. Discuss the reality of patients taking their own medications in long-term care facilities.
- Invite a home care supervisor into class to discuss the role of the medication aide. If the supervisor does not give medications, discuss how to supervise the patient as he or she takes medications. (Many Certified Medication Aides are Certified Nurse Aides also.)
- If possible, show a film about older patients. Show how the pharmacokinetics of aging affect their reaction to the effects of drugs. Ask the students to summarize the material in relation to their working with older patients and giving them medications. They can do this in different ways—writing papers, demonstrating body changes using posters or simulated organs, or acting out adverse drug effects.
- Ask a gerontologist or a nurse specializing in gerontology to talk to the class. Ask the students to prepare a list of questions regarding the number of doctors, pharmacists, and family members involved in older patients' care. How can students cooperate in the care so patients are not abusing drugs?
- Have students write a paper or discuss in class why almost all older patients are special-risk patients (organ impairment, arthritis, other common diseases of the older patient).
- Assign the students to research the present attitudes about the aging population as compared to attitudes some years ago. What percentage of hospital patients are over 65? Will this be changing? What are the government, state, or local authorities doing to help this group of patients?
- Ask students to complete the Chapter 20 Review. Discuss answers, clearing up any misconceptions students may have. Review any material students had difficulty with.
- Administer and grade the Chapter 20 Test in this Instructor's Manual.

Critical Thinking Activities

1. Discuss why drug absorption and distribution are slower and less predictable in elderly patients.
2. Develop a plan for administering medications to elderly patients.

Answers to Chapter 20 Review

1. Branch of medicine that deals with diseases and disorders of old age.
2. Study of the problems of the elderly.
3. A number of different drugs used by a patient who may have several different health problems.
4. Over the counter, available without a prescription.
5. The skin becomes thinner and dryer and loses its suppleness. The fatty layer under the skin disappears, causing wrinkles and folds and giving less protection against cold and injury. Bruising is more common. Spots of color appear on the skin, and small vessels are likely to burst, causing "spiders." Sweating decreases, and there is less blood flow to the skin. Elderly

bedridden patients are at a high risk of developing decubitous ulcers, or pressure sores.

6. The heart pumps less forcefully and pumps less blood with each beat, even though the number of beats per minute increases. The heart has less ability to gear up for action when the body is under stress. Various parts of the heart and the blood vessels lose their elasticity, and fatty substances may be deposited on the inner layers of arteries. These deposits give more resistance to the pumping action of the heart, so hypertension may develop. There is less blood flow to all parts of the body.
7. Collagen settles in the lungs, lessening their ability to expand. Along with a reduced flow of blood to the lungs, this makes respiration less efficient, and not as much oxygen is supplied to the body. In order to make up for this deficiency, an older person must breathe faster than the normal 16–20 times per minute. Breathing is also shallower.
8. Brain cells die and there is less blood flow to the brain, affecting memory and the ability to make decisions. Confused thinking and changes in personality can result from the poor supply of oxygen to the brain.
9. Sensory messages do not come in strong and clear. The eyes have a harder time adjusting to changes in light. The ears do not hear the higher sounds, and hearing aids may be needed. Taste and smell are dulled so that eating is less pleasurable. The sense of touch is dulled.
10. The secretions and muscular movements of the digestive tract slow down, and the elderly produce less stomach acid than normal. These changes make food harder to digest and slower to move through the system. Indigestion and constipation are common problems. If teeth are lost or inflamed, eating may become difficult or uncomfortable. The absorption of nutrients from the intestines is less efficient, so nutrition may be affected.
11. There is less blood flow to the kidneys, and there are changes within the kidneys themselves. They do not filter the blood as efficiently, so wastes are excreted more slowly. They cannot adapt as quickly as before to changes in the fluid/electrolyte balance.
12. All the glands secrete less of their hormones. As a result, body cell metabolism is not as well regulated and the body cannot react as quickly to stress. Most elderly persons develop some degree of diabetes.
13. Usually after age 48 or 50 females no longer menstruate or conceive babies. In both men and women, sex hormone production decreases, with resulting physical changes. However, because attitudes and emotions, not just hormones, determine sexual enjoyment, older people can still enjoy an active sex life.
14. Muscles lose strength and flexibility. There is also an increase in the percentage of body fat, replacing muscle. The bones become lighter and more porous, so they are more apt to fracture easily and heal slowly. Ligaments and joints are subject to stiffening and thickening. Diseases of bones, joints, and ligaments are more common.
15. The dose is usually smaller and given less often to make up for changes in absorption, distribution, metabolism, and excretion in the elderly. This is the general rule, but drug treatment must be individualized for each patient.
16. They differ because people age at different rates, and different body systems age at different times. This means that each man's medication therapy must be individualized according to the systems that have aged the most.
17. There has been a gradual loss of elasticity in the lungs because of deposits of the protein collagen. This means less oxygen intake with each

breath, so Ms. Peach must breathe more often to get the same amount of oxygen as before.

18. His confusion might be due to the effects of some of the medications on his nervous system. Or there might be a lack of oxygen in the brain due to poor circulation that comes with aging.
19. Let Mrs. Nimitz participate in her own medication plan, pour her own water if she can, and take her own pills under supervision. You will explain the procedure and the reason for medication so that Mrs. Nimitz is fully informed.
20. Poor liver function would slow down the metabolism of the drugs, and poor kidney function would slow excretion. The adverse reactions to look out for would be drug cumulating and possibly toxicity.
21. Inform her that both aspirin and tranquilizers could be dangerous while she is on anticoagulants because of drug interactions. She should turn over the medications until the doctor says that they are safe to use. She should discard the tranquilizers, since they were prescribed for her sister and not for her.
22. Putting off the charting until later might lead to medication errors. For example, another staff member may give a patient a p.r.n. medication even though you gave it an hour ago.
23. He may have a hearing problem. You could try speaking slowly and clearly, standing so that he can see your face (to read lips). If that does not work, you might try writing down the instructions for him (in large, clear letters). There is also the possibility that he may not understand English, so you might need someone to translate.
24. Explain what the medications are and what they do. Sit with Ms. Brill to gain her confidence and ease her fears. If she still refuses, do not force her to take the medications, but inform the nurse in charge and await further instructions.

Chapter 20 Test Answers

1. a	2. b	3. d	4. c	5. b	6. d	7. d
8. d	9. d	10. a	11. c	12. d	13. a	14. b
15. b	16. T	17. F	18. F	19. T	20. F	21. T
22. T	23. T	24. F	25. F			

Name ______________________ Date ____________________ Class ____________

Chapter 1 Test

Circle the letter of the best choice.

1. Pharmacology is the study of
   a. the medical field.
   b. the art of preparing drug compounds.
   c. drugs.
   d. the health sciences.
2. Pharmacodynamics is the study of
   a. the interactions between drugs and the body.
   b. drug sources.
   c. the medical field.
   d. the diseases of the body.
3. The study of how body parts work is called
   a. physiology.
   b. psychology.
   c. pharmaceuticals.
   d. pharmacy.
4. Anatomy is the study of
   a. the functions of the body parts.
   b. the structure of the body parts.
   c. the mind.
   d. drugs used in the human body.
5. Which of the following is not a drug reference?
   a. *PDR®*
   b. USP/NF
   c. medical dictionary
   d. AHFS
6. Chemical synthesis/genetic engineering refers to
   a. extracting drugs from plants.
   b. extracting drugs from animals.
   c. administering drugs to laboratory animals.
   d. creating drugs in the laboratory.
7. A drug may have several product names but only one
   a. brand name.
   b. OTC name.
   c. proprietary name.
   d. generic name.
8. The drug name owned by the manufacturer is called the
   a. trade name.
   b. product name.
   c. brand name.
   d. all of the above.

9. The generic name is usually the same as the
   a. official name.
   b. brand name.
   c. chemical name.
   d. trade name.
10. The drug name that describes the structure of the drug compound is the
   a. official name.
   b. trade name.
   c. chemical name.
   d. proprietary name.
11. Rules that ensure uniform strength, quality, and purity of drugs are called
   a. drug standards.
   b. drug references.
   c. drug laws.
   d. drug specifications.
12. If you needed to identify a little pink tablet that your patient brought from home in an unlabeled bottle, which drug reference would you use?
   a. USP/NF
   b. nursing journals
   c. *PDR*®
   d. Hospital Formulary
13. If you have a question about how to administer a particular drug and know only the drug's generic name, where can you find drugs listed by generic names?
   a. *PDR*®
   b. AHFS
   c. USP/NF
   d. all of the above

Read the reprinted section of the *PDR*®. Then answer questions 14 and 15.

Esidrix® ℞
(ess´adricks)
(hydrochlorothiazide USP)

Indications and Usage
Hypertension: In the management of hypertension either as the sole therapeutic agent or to enhance the effects of other antihypertensive drugs in the more severe forms of hypertension.
Edema: As adjunctive therapy in edema associated with congestive heart failure, hepatic cirrhosis, and corticosteroid and estrogen therapy.
Esidrix has also been found useful in edema due to various forms of renal dysfunction, such as the nephrotic syndrome, acute glomerulonephritis, and chronic renal failure.
Usage in Pregnancy: The routine use of diuretics in an otherwise healthy woman is inappropriate and exposes mother and fetus to unnecessary hazard. Diuretics do not prevent development of toxemia of pregnancy, and there is no satisfactory evidence that they are useful in the treatment of developed toxemia.

14. *Esidrix* is used in drug therapy for
    a. hypertension.
    b. pregnancy.
    c. hypertension and edema.
    d. hypertension, edema, and pregnancy.
15. The generic name for *Esidrix* is
    a. hypertension.
    b. hydrochlorothiazide.
    c. hydrochloric acid.
    d. hematology.
16. Which is not true of the Controlled Substances Act?
    a. It is enforced by the DEA.
    b. It regulates the manufacture and sale of narcotics and dangerous drugs.
    c. It regulates prescription drugs and cosmetics.
    d. It has five schedules of drugs with special restrictions.
17. The first drug law passed in the United States was the
    a. Pure Food and Drug Act.
    b. Controlled Substances Act.
    c. Food, Drug, and Cosmetic Act.
    d. Drug Enforcement Act.
18. Examples of drugs made from plant sources are
    a. iron and salt.
    b. heparin and insulin.
    c. digitalis and opium.
    d. sulfa drugs and hydroxyurea.
19. Pharmacology includes the study of
    a. dosage and administration routes.
    b. drug sources and ingredients.
    c. normal and abnormal effects of drugs.
    d. all of the above.
20. Medications are administered to
    a. prevent, diagnose, treat, and cure disease.
    b. prevent pregnancy.
    c. maintain good health.
    d. all of the above.
21. Drug references
    a. are always up to date.
    b. need to be updated regularly.
    c. are usually written in clear and simple language.
    d. are of no use to the health worker.
22. Controlled substances
    a. can be abused or cause dependence.
    b. have limits on who can buy and sell them.
    c. must have the physician's DEA number on the prescription.
    d. all of the above.

23. Drugs that can be bought and sold without any special restrictions are
    a. OTC drugs.
    b. prescription drugs.
    c. pharmacy drugs.
    d. controlled substances.
24. A person who gives medications needs to know and follow the drug laws
    a. to live up to the responsibilities of his or her job.
    b. to set a good example for the patient.
    c. to avoid fines and imprisonment.
    d. all of the above.

Name ______________________ Date ____________________ Class ____________

Chapter 2 Test

Circle the letter of the best choice.

1. Pharmacokinetics is the study of
   a. how the body handles a drug.
   b. the best ways to prepare drugs.
   c. the signs and symptoms of disease.
   d. none of the above.

2. Which of the following do not affect drug action?
   a. absorption and distribution
   b. metabolism and excretion
   c. sensation and perception
   d. condition of the liver and kidneys

3. In drug therapy, drugs are usually given because of their
   a. therapeutic effects.
   b. side effects.
   c. adverse effects.
   d. synergistic effects.

4. Drug dependence is
   a. a therapeutic effect of a drug.
   b. a mental or physical craving for a drug.
   c. abuse of a drug.
   d. an emotional reaction to a drug.

5. Which of these drugs are commonly abused?
   a. narcotics and stimulants
   b. sedatives and tranquilizers
   c. marijuana and alcohol
   d. all of the above

6. A patient shows signs of drowsiness and extreme euphoria. On examination, you discover a very slow heartbeat and needle marks on the patient's arm. You think the person may be taking drugs for nonmedical reasons. You would tell your supervisor you suspect
   a. allergy.
   b. synergism.
   c. drug abuse.
   d. antagonism.

7. The health care worker's responsibility in adverse reaction is to
   a. reduce the dose.
   b. increase the dose.
   c. immediately call the nurse in charge or the supervisor.
   d. change the medication.

8. The health care worker's responsibility when caring for a drug abuse patient is to
   a. decide when a patient is abusing drugs.
   b. notify the supervisor when drug abuse is suspected.
   c. administer drugs as requested by the patient.
   d. notify the patient's family.
9. Drug action is
   a. the psychological effect of the drug.
   b. the way in which the drug affects the chemistry of body cells.
   c. an unusual response to a drug.
   d. the main reason for not giving drugs.
10. Drug effects are
   a. ways of administering drugs.
   b. examples of drug misuse.
   c. the way a drug interacts with body cells.
   d. physical changes in the body as a result of drug action.
11. A skin lotion is applied to dry skin for a(n)
   a. systemic effect.
   b. adverse effect.
   c. local effect.
   d. unusual effect.
12. Withdrawal symptoms include
   a. euphoria and excitement.
   b. coughing.
   c. feelings of relief.
   d. nausea and sweating.
13. Your patient has just started taking several new medications at once. You will observe for
   a. synergism and antagonism.
   b. allergy.
   c. tolerance and cumulation.
   d. all of the above.
14. Drug action is affected by many factors. All of the following affect drug action except
   a. the patient's intelligence.
   b. the patient's size and age.
   c. other drugs the patient is taking.
   d. time and route of administration.
15. The four main drug actions are slowing cell functions, destroying cells, replacing substances, and
   a. removing wastes.
   b. speeding up cell processes.
   c. antagonizing the cells.
   d. potentiating the cells.

16. A drug overdose can lead to
    a. toxicity.
    b. sensitivity.
    c. withdrawal symptoms.
    d. all of the above.
17. Health care workers can prevent drug abuse by
    a. giving patients controlled substances as needed.
    b. keeping medications locked up when not in use.
    c. using amphetamines to stay awake on the night shift.
    d. all of the above.
18. Because of a disease condition, a patient's liver cannot metabolize drugs very quickly. They begin to collect in the patient's body, so you see a stronger effect after each dose. This is an example of
    a. cumulation.
    b. synergism.
    c. drug dependence.
    d. tolerance.
19. A decreased physiological response to repeated administrations of a drug is
    a. idiosyncrasy.
    b. toxicity.
    c. tolerance.
    d. cumulation.

Match the terms in the right column to the best description in the left column.

______	20. Drugs leaving the body	a. absorption
______	21. Drugs entering the bloodstream from the site of administration	b. biotransformation
______	22. Drugs passing into cells and into spaces between cells	c. distribution
______	23. Drugs being broken down into substances that can be excreted	d. excretion
______	24. Drugs that circulate throughout the body	e. local
______	25. Drugs that affect only the area where they are administered	f. systemic

Name ______________________ Date ____________________ Class ____________

Chapter 3 Test

Circle the letter of the best choice.

1. The metric system is based on units of
   a. 6.
   b. 10.
   c. 25.
   d. 60.

2. Abbreviations for apothecary units of measurement include
   a. gr, m, oz, dr.
   b. L, mg, cc, kg.
   c. gtt, tsp, oz, pt.
   d. in, ft, yd, mi.

3. Which is the correct way to abbreviate "one and one-half grains"?
   a. 1.5 g
   b. $1\frac{1}{2}$ gr
   c. gr $\overline{\text{iss}}$
   d. b and c

4. One thousandth of a liter is a
   a. microliter.
   b. miniliter.
   c. pentameter.
   d. milliliter.

5. One cubic centimeter is the same as
   a. 1 grain.
   b. 1 milliliter.
   c. 1 liter.
   d. 1 ounce.

6. A patient was given 10 gtt of potassium iodide at bedtime; 10 gtt means
   a. 10 drops.
   b. 10 milliliters.
   c. 1 ounce.
   d. 1 dram.

7. A patient was given a liter of saline solution intravenously. A liter is about the same as
   a. 500 cubic centimeters.
   b. 1 cup.
   c. 1 pint.
   d. 1 quart.

8. The label says "*Nitro-Bid* 2.5 mg." This shows the drug is weighed in metric units. If you changed the dosage to apothecary units, you would state the dosage in
   a. grains.
   b. grams.
   c. milliliters.
   d. drops.
9. Medicine ordered from the pharmacy and received is marked 0.5 g. This is the same as
   a. 50 grains.
   b. 500 grains.
   c. 500 milligrams.
   d. 5 cubic centimeters.
10. 75 mg is the same as
    a. 0.75 gram.
    b. 7.5 grams.
    c. 0.075 gram.
    d. 7500 grams.
11. For an infection of the respiratory tract, the doctor orders 400,000 units of *V-Cillin K* every 6 hours. From the pharmacy you receive tablets that each contain 200,000 units of the drug. How many tablets will you administer every 6 hours?
    a. one
    b. two
    c. three
    d. one-half
12. A patient with anxiety is to receive 20 mg of *Librium* 4 times a day. You have 5-mg *Librium* tablets from the pharmacy. How many of these tablets should you give the patient for one dose?
    a. one
    b. two
    c. three
    d. four
13. A very young child needs a liquid form of acetaminophen, a pain reliever. You have a bottle labeled "Acetaminophen 2 gr per teaspoon." The doctor has ordered 1 gr per dose. How much do you give?
    a. 2 tsp
    b. 1 tsp
    c. $\frac{1}{2}$ tsp
    d. $\frac{1}{4}$ tsp
14. The pharmacy has sent up *Lasix* for a patient. The bottle is labeled "10 mg per ml." The physician's order calls for a dose of 40 mg twice a day. How much is the correct dose to give the patient?
    a. 4 ml
    b. 0.25 ml
    c. 1 ml
    d. 4 tsp

15. The order for nitroglycerin states 1/150 gr subl. p.r.n. for angina. The pharmacy sends up sublingual tablets that contain 0.4 mg per tablet. How many tablets would you give the patient at one time?
    a. $\frac{1}{4}$ tablet
    b. $\frac{1}{2}$ tablet
    c. 1 tablet
    d. 2 tablets
16. When calculating a child's dose, it is assumed that the usual adult dose is for a person who weighs
    a. 125 lb.
    b. 150 lb.
    c. 175 lb.
    d. 160 lb.
17. Chloral hydrate comes in 5 gr, 10 gr, and 15 gr capsules. In order to give a patient 900 mg of the drug, you would give
    a. one 5 gr capsule.
    b. one 10 gr capsule.
    c. one 15 gr capsule.
    d. two 10 gr capsules.
18. The doctor ordered one teaspoon of *Pepto-Bismol* for your patient. You do not have a teaspoon on hand to measure it, but you do have a medicine glass marked in milliliters. So you give the patient
    a. 5 ml.
    b. 8 ml.
    c. 15 ml.
    d. 24 ml.
19. Ampicillin is sent up from the pharmacy in 100 mg scored tablets. The doctor has ordered 250 mg for a patient to be given 4 times a day. For one dose you would give the patient
    a. 2 tablets.
    b. $2\frac{1}{2}$ tablets.
    c. 3 tablets.
    d. $3\frac{1}{2}$ tablets.
20. In dosage calculation, a "child" is someone who is
    a. under 16 years of age.
    b. under 10 years of age.
    c. between 5 and 15 years of age.
    d. under $12\frac{1}{2}$ years.
21. After calculating a dose of medicine for a patient, you feel unsure about the dose you got. You feel it might be too high. You should
    a. give the medication and hope for the best.
    b. keep quiet about it—the supervisor might think you aren't very bright.
    c. assume you did it correctly, because you don't make mistakes often.
    d. ask the nurse in charge to check your calculation.

22. A young child has a temperature of 40°C. You convert the temperature to _____ °F and call the doctor.

a. 99.4° F

b. 100.8° F

c. 102.6° F

d. 104° F

23. A patient has a temperature of 101.2° F also has temperature of ____ ° C.

a. 32° C

b. 38.4° C

c. 52.8° C

d. 74° C

Match these equivalents.

______	24 0.1 mg	a.	1 gr
______	25. 1 mg	b.	1/600 gr
______	26. 60 mg	c.	15 gr
______	27. 1 g	d.	1/60 gr

Solve these problems.

28. $\frac{500 \text{ cc}}{5 \text{ hr.}} \times \frac{15 \text{ gtt}}{1 \text{ cc}} \times \frac{1 \text{ hr}}{60 \text{ min}} =$

29. $\frac{240 \text{ cc}}{6 \text{ hr}} \times \frac{60 \text{ micro gtt}}{1 \text{ cc}} \times \frac{1 \text{ hr}}{60 \text{ min}} =$

Name ______________________ Date ____________________ Class ____________

Chapter 4 Test

Circle the letter of the best choice.

1. Alcohol solutions such as spirits, elixirs, fluidextracts, and tinctures should be kept in a
   a. light place.
   b. tightly capped bottle.
   c. suspension chamber.
   d. all of the above.
2. When measuring fluidextracts, it is best to use a
   a. teaspoon.
   b. tablespoon.
   c. glass.
   d. medicine dropper.
3. Suspensions such as magmas, emulsions, and gels
   a. should be shaken after use.
   b. need not be shaken.
   c. should be shaken before use.
   d. should be shaken only if ordered to do so.
4. A liniment is administered
   a. by rubbing it into the skin.
   b. by patting it on the skin.
   c. subcutaneously.
   d. by instillation.
5. Examples of solid and semisolid forms of medications are
   a. tinctures, elixirs, spirits, fluidextracts.
   b. suppositories, capsules, tablets, dry extracts.
   c. ointments, gels, magmas, mixtures.
   d. suspensions and solutions.
6. A lotion should not be
   a. rubbed into the skin.
   b. patted on the skin.
   c. shaken before use.
   d. used to lubricate the skin.
7. An ointment can be instilled in the eyes only if
   a. it is shaken before use.
   b. the ingredients are labeled.
   c. it is labeled "Sterile—Ophthalmic Use."
   d. it is a gel.
8. Which is not true of a delayed-release tablet?
   a. effects last for many hours
   b. medication layers dissolve at different times
   c. it contains many doses of medicine
   d. it can be crushed and mixed with applesauce

9. Another name for delayed-release capsules is
   a. troches.
   b. magmas.
   c. emulsions.
   d. sustained-release.

10. Enteric-coated capsules or tablets dissolve in the
    a. mouth.
    b. stomach.
    c. intestines.
    d. rectum.

11. Troches and lozenges dissolve in the
    a. mouth.
    b. stomach.
    c. intestines.
    d. rectum.

12. An example of sublingual administration is
    a. a capsule swallowed with water.
    b. a tablet that dissolves under the tongue.
    c. a cream gently rubbed into the skin.
    d. an injection under the skin.

13. Suppositories are never administered
    a. rectally.
    b. vaginally.
    c. parenterally.
    d. into the urethra.

14. An example of inhalation administration is
    a. breathing a mist containing an asthma reliever.
    b. sucking a mentholated cough drop.
    c. spraying a topical anesthetic on a burn.
    d. swabbing a mucous membrane.

15. Parenteral administration can be performed by
    a. physicians only.
    b. nurses only.
    c. nurse aides only.
    d. any medical personnel specially trained and certified to give injections.

16. A patient is unable to take large capsules and tablets. The usual procedure in such cases is to dissolve the medication in food or drink. Which of the following substances would be appropriate for dissolving a delayed-release cold tablet?
    a. applesauce
    b. mashed potatoes
    c. milk
    d. none of the above

17. A medication order must always be
    a. stated verbally.
    b. written.
    c. signed by the physician.
    d. typewritten.

18. Medication orders for outpatients are written on a
    a. doctor's order sheet.
    b. prescription blank.
    c. pharmacy requisition.
    d. controlled-substance form.

19. A physician is working at a clinic across town today and wants to call in an order for a patient at your facility. Who should write down the verbal order taken over the phone?
    a. only the nurse in charge
    b. any health worker
    c. no one; phone orders are not allowed
    d. depends on state law and the policy of your facility

20. Medication orders do not usually include
    a. the name of the drug.
    b. the date.
    c. the patient's full name.
    d. the patient's room and bed number.

21. Which item tells you something about the dosage?
    a. q.2h.
    b. 50 mg
    c. 2 tablets
    d. all of the above

22. You are instructed to administer a medication to a patient at 0800, 1200, 1600, and 2000 hours. This is the same as
    a. 8 P.M., midnight, 6 A.M., and 10 A.M.
    b. 8 A.M., 12 noon, 4 P.M., and 8 P.M.
    c. 8 A.M., 12 noon, 5 P.M., and 9 P.M.
    d. 8 P.M., midnight, 4 A.M., and 8 A.M.

23. Prescriptions for Schedule II controlled substances
    a. may be refilled up to 5 times.
    b. do not need to be signed.
    c. must include the doctor's DEA number.
    d. must show the name of the drug on the label.

24. Automatic-stop orders are
    a. to be given immediately and only once.
    b. self-terminating orders.
    c. given for controlled substances only.
    d. all of the above.

25. The doctor's order book is smudged and the patient's medication order is hard to read. You should
    a. refuse to give the medication.
    b. look up the drug in a drug reference.
    c. ask the physician to repeat or rewrite the order.
    d. use your judgment as to the correct dosage.
26. Abbreviations for forms of medication include
    a. B.I.D., h.s., A.M., P.M.
    b. sp., tr., fld.ext., oint.
    c. stat, P.R.N., s.o.s., q.s.
    d. subl., SL, r., IV, ID.
27. Medication abbreviations for how often a drug is given include
    a. OD, OS, OU, ophth.
    b. buc., ID, hypo., subl., SL.
    c. supp., ext., syr.
    d. P.R.N., Q.H., Q.O.D., Q.I.D.
28. Which abbreviations are most likely to be found on an order for eye medication?
    a. OD, OU, OS, ophth.
    b. IM, IV, ID, SQ
    c. n.p.o., stat., "O," h.s.
    d. B.I.D., T.I.D., Q.I.D., Q.O.D.
29. A patient with angina is taking the medication *Nitro-Bid.* The doctor's order sheet says: *Nitro-Bid* caps 250 mg b.i.d. Each capsule contains 250 mg. What will you administer?
    a. one capsule before meals
    b. one capsule 2 times a day
    c. one capsule 3 times a day
    d. two capsules once a day
30. Drugs can be injected into the vein via
    a. a volume controlled chamber.
    b. a heparin lock.
    c. special entry areas in IV tubing.
    d. a patient controlled pump (PCA).

A patient is being treated for a painful skin disease. His body is covered with sores and he has fever, nausea, and chills. His physician orders ampicillin to stop the infection and *Dimetane* to dry up the sores. The physician orders chloral hydrate, a sedative, to help the patient sleep. Two days later, the physician orders *Maalox,* an antacid, because the patient has an upset stomach as a side effect of the *Dimetane.*

Read through the physician's order sheet. Then answer questions 31 through 35.

31. Which drug is to be given at bedtime?
    a. chloral hydrate
    b. *Dimetane*
    c. amoxicillin
    d. *Maalox*

32. Which medication should be given 3 times a day?
    a. chloral hydrate
    b. ampicillin
    c. *Dimetane*
    d. *Maalox*
33. Which medication can the nurse decide to give when the patient seems to need it?
    a. chloral hydrate
    b. *Dimetane*
    c. ampicillin
    d. *Maalox*
34. "Amoxicillin 250 mg p.o. q.8h. × 10 days" is a
    a. standing order.
    b. automatic stop order (ASO).
    c. stat order.
    d. P.R.N. order.
35. "*Maalox* 2 tsp p.r.n." is a
    a. standing order.
    b. self-terminating order.
    c. automic stop order.
    d. stat order.
36. Drugs are delivered from the pharmacy in
    a. initial dose and maintenance dose packages.
    b. big dose and small dose packages.
    c. clinical dose and pharmacy dose packages.
    d. multiple-dose and single-dose packages.
37. Unit dose packages
    a. cannot be returned for credit.
    b. are more likely to involve medication errors.
    c. are safer because there is no drug handling involved.
    d. must be disposed of if some doses are left over.
38. Store all medications in the
    a. patient's night table.
    b. medicine room.
    c. locked nurse's desk.
    d. linen supply closet.
39. You are wondering whether a certain drug needs to be refrigerated. The best place to look for the answer is
    a. in a drug reference book.
    b. on the doctor's order sheet.
    c. on a list posted on the refrigerator door.
    d. on a note from the pharmacist.

40. Order stock supply drugs
    a. before they are used up.
    b. after they are used up.
    c. at the beginning of each month.
    d. on the next shift.

41. You prepared a dose of milk of magnesia for a patient, but before you could give it to the patient, he had an emergency and was moved into the intensive care unit. What should you do with his dose of milk of magnesia?
    a. keep it on the medicine cart, but not in the supply bottle
    b. pour it back in the bottle to avoid wasting it
    c. save it for another patient at their next scheduled medication time
    d. dispose of it in the proper manner

42. Keeping the medication room clean helps to
    a. prevent medication errors.
    b. keep out unauthorized personnel.
    c. keep out the patients.
    d. prevent contamination of the unit doses.

43. To find the correct way to dispose of any drug
    a. check with the doctor.
    b. check the policy of your facility.
    c. check the Kardex.
    d. check a drug reference.

44. In a hospital, medication orders are usually copied onto
    a. a patient history sheet.
    b. medication records.
    c. nurse's notes.
    d. both b and c.

45. The Kardex includes information about the
    a. history of the patient's disease symptoms.
    b. daily medications and treatments ordered by the doctor.
    c. progress of the patient.
    d. patient's family situation.

46. A medicine card is unreadable because medication was accidentally spilled on it. You would
    a. copy the information over.
    b. give the drug dosage as you remember it from yesterday.
    c. not give the medicine at all.
    d. do the best you can to read through the spillage.

47. When setting up medication, it is important to notice
    a. the expiration date on the package.
    b. changes in texture, smell, or color of the drug.
    c. the name of the drug printed on the package.
    d. all of the above.

48. To divide a scored tablet evenly, use
    a. your thumbnails.
    b. the edge of a knife.
    c. the back of a spoon.
    d. a medicine cup.

49. Controlled substances are counted
    a. once a day.
    b. during the night shift and afternoon shift only.
    c. and signed for at the beginning of each shift.
    d. and signed for sometime during each shift.

50. The patient chart is
    a. a means of communication.
    b. used only in offices and clinics.
    c. not acceptable in court cases.
    d. a record of controlled substance use.

51. A chart is a record of events in
    a. the health care worker's daily routine.
    b. the hospital unit.
    c. the patient's care treatment.
    d. the jobs of the health care team.

52. A patient was in the X-ray department when the time came for her last medication. As a result, you could not give her the prescribed dose of medicine. You must tell the nurse in charge about the missed medication and also
    a. tell the doctor.
    b. record it on an "incident form."
    c. chart it on the nurse's notes and the medication record.
    d. give the patient a double dose the next time.

53. The basic rules and regulations of medication administration
    a. change according to who is receiving the medication.
    b. change according to the type of drug.
    c. change according to who gives the medication.
    d. never change.

54. When setting up medications, read the label at least
    a. 1 time.
    b. 2 times.
    c. 3 times.
    d. 4 times.

55. If you make a medication error, your best course of action is to
    a. forget it; you will do better next time.
    b. report it and review the events that led up to the error.
    c. ask the nurse in charge to remind you to pass meds.
    d. tell the patient to put the call light on at medication time.

Questions 56 through 60 are to be answered using the accompanying Kardex sheet, medication record, and nurses' notes.

56. According to the Kardex, the last dose of *Chloromycetin* ointment is to be given at
    a. 0900 on May 11.
    b. 01200 on April 25.
    c. 1800 on May 11.
    d. 1500 on April 25.

Questions 57 through 60 are to be answered directly on the appropriate form.

57. Carol Theiss is in the Physical Therapy Department at 1700 on April 30. You are unable to give her the scheduled dose of *Dilantin.* Chart this fact on the nurses' notes and the medication record.
58. Carol refuses her 1800 application of eye ointment. She says it causes a burning sensation in her eyes. The date is 4/30/98. Chart the facts on the nurses' notes and the medication record.
59. It is 1000 on May 1 and Carol Theiss is asking for a pill that will ease her headache. Check the Kardex to see if she is allowed to have one. Then chart it on the nurses' notes and the medication record.
60. It is 2000 on May 2. Carol wants a laxative to ease her constipation. Check the Kardex. If she is allowed to have a laxative, chart it on the nurses' notes and the medication record.

When you have passed this mastery test, sign up for a performance test on

- transcribing medication orders.
- writing down verbal medication orders.
- counting controlled substances.
- recording the use of controlled substances.
- setting up medications on a tray with medicine cards.
- dispensing unit-dose medications from a cart.
- filling out an incident report form.
- dispensing unit-dose medications from a cart.
- filling out an incident report form.

PRN MEDICATIONS

ROOM NO. 124		PT. NAME Carol Theiss		
ANALGESICS	SCHEDULE	NO. OF UNITS SUPPLIED	MDU / ONE TIME DOSES	QUAN.
Tylenol GR10 PO	Q 4h PRN			
LAXATIVES				
MOM 30 ML	PRN			
Nausea				
MISC				
SEDATIVES				
Dalmane MG. PO	HS PRN			

Number 07186 **Scheduled Medications** Dischge. Date ________ By ____________

Period & Doses 10:30-7:30	7:30-10:30	Medication	Rt.	Dose	Schedule	Doses Supplied First	Last	Omitted doses /Spec. Inst.	Total Units
		Dilantin	p.o.	100 mg.	T.I.D.	4/25			
		Chloromycetin	op.		q. 3h.	4/25	5/11	DC 2000	

Diagnosis SEIZURES		**Allergies**	**Age** 24
Rm. 124	**Name** CAROL THEISS		**IV**

UNIT DOSE MEDICATION RECORD

SCHEDULED DRUGS

START / STOP	RN OK	MEDICATIONS AND DOSE	RTE.	SCED	DATE 4/30/xx	DATE 5/1/xx	DATE 5/2/xx	DATE 5/3/xx
4/25	D.V.	Dilantin 100mg.	p.o.	t.i.d.	DW ~~0900~~ - EH ~~1300~~ - YN (1700)	0900-1300-1700	0900-1300-1700	0900-1300-1700
4/25 / 5/11		Chloromycetin	Op	q.3h.	DW ~~0900~~ - EH ~~1200~~ - EH ~~1500~~ - YN (1800)	0900-1200-1500-1800	0900-1200-1500-1800	0900-1200-1500-1800
		ophth. oint.						
4/25		Tylenol gr X p.r.n.	p.o.	q.4h.				
		for headache						
		Milk of Mag. 30ml	p.o.					
		h.s. p.r.n. for						
		constipation						

PRN

06-0535-2.2-77

Signatures

Doug Waters

Ellen Houck

Your Name

NURSES' NOTES

Family Name	First Name	Attending Physician	Room No.	Hosp. No.
Theiss,	Carol	Dr. Meese	124	54-783

Date	Time	REMARKS - TREATMENT	Nurse's Signature

Name ________________ Date ________________ Class ________________

Chapter 5 Test

Circle the letter of the best choice.

1. A deficiency of vitamin D causes
   a. night blindness.
   b. pellegra.
   c. rickets.
   d. pernicious anemia.
2. Vitamin C helps
   a. wounds heal properly.
   b. breakdown fats.
   c. improve vision.
   d. heart function.
3. The recommended number of daily servings for vegetables is
   a. 6–11.
   b. 1–2.
   c. 4.
   d. 3–5.
4. Taking too much vitamin A results in
   a. nausea, vomiting, and abdominal pain.
   b. a rapid heart rate.
   c. jaundice.
   d. a urinary tract infection.
5. Vitamins are
   a. inorganic elements essential to the body.
   b. solutions that carry an electrical charge.
   c. organic elements essential for normal metabolism.
   d. compounds that do not contain carbon.
6. The vitamin necessary for healthy bones and teeth is
   a. D.
   b. E.
   c. K.
   d. B_1.
7. The vitamin necessary for vision is
   a. C.
   b. D.
   c. A.
   d. B_6.
8. A water-soluble vitamin is
   a. A.
   b. C.
   c. D.
   d. K.

9. The recommended daily allowance (RDA) for vitamins and minerals is
   a. determined by an individual's illness.
   b. based on the average normal, healthy adult.
   c. different every day.
   d. established by vitamin and mineral supplements only.
10. Examples of macrominerals are
    a. calcium and potassium.
    b. zinc and cobalt.
    c. iron and manganese.
    d. fluoride and copper.
11. An example of an electrolyte is
    a. vitamin A.
    b. iron.
    c. vitamin D.
    d. sodium.
12. The herb that maintains a healthy urinary tract is
    a. cranberry.
    b. St. John's wort.
    c. ginkgo.
    d. elderberry.
13. The mineral responsible for the development of the thyroid gland is
    a. iron.
    b. calcium.
    c. iodine.
    d. sodium.
14. The function of vitamin K is
    a. never conduction.
    b. formation of prothrombin for blood clotting.
    c. maintenance of healthy bones and teeth.
    d. formation of collagen.
15. A major source of iron is
    a. strawberries.
    b. liver.
    c. pickles.
    d. raisins.
16. Which vitamin is found in sunlight?
    a. A
    b. B
    c. C
    d. D
17. The vitamin manufactured in the intestinal tract is
    a. B_1.
    b. B_3.
    c. C.
    d. K.

18. A deficiency of vitamin B_1 causes
    a. tingling and numbness in extremities.
    b. cracks around corners of mouth.
    c. anemia.
    d. loose teeth.
19. The mineral used in a patient taking diuretics is
    a. calcium.
    b. iron.
    c. potassium.
    d. phosphorus.
20. The mineral that causes serious cardiac changes is
    a. magnesium.
    b. potassium.
    c. calcium.
    d. iodine.
21. The mineral that causes constipation and black stools is
    a. zinc.
    b. sodium.
    c. copper.
    d. iron.
22. A drug that is made from the foxglove plant is
    a. *Lanoxin.*
    b. *Oncovin.*
    c. *Velban.*
    d. *Serpasil.*
23. The popular herb taken to promote a positive feeling of well-being is
    a. green tea.
    b. St. John's wort.
    c. cat's claw.
    d. valerian root.
24. An adequate intake of vitamin A prevents
    a. osteomalacia.
    b. scurvy.
    c. pernicious anemia.
    d. nightblindness.
25. Milk and milk products are the major source of
    a. iodine.
    b. copper.
    c. calcium.
    d. potassium.
26. Aloe vera is a common herb used for
    a. its antioxidant properties.
    b. mild sedation.
    c. the acceleration of wound healing.
    d. vasodilation.

Name ______________________ Date ____________________ Class ____________

Chapter 6 Test

Circle the letter of the best choice.

1. An agent that inhibits the growth or multiplication of bacteria is
   a. disinfectant.
   b. bactericidal.
   c. antibody.
   d. bacteriostatic.

2. Tiny one-celled plants and animals are
   a. leukocytes.
   b. inoculation.
   c. penicillinase.
   d. microorganisms.

3. The body's ability to resist damage from pathogens is
   a. immunity.
   b. aseptic.
   c. immunization.
   d. superinfection.

4. A substance produced by the body to kill a specific type of microorganism is a(n)
   a. antibody.
   b. antiseptic.
   c. pathogen.
   d. leukocyte.

5. The white blood cells that defend the body against invading microorganisms are
   a. autoclaves.
   b. antibodies.
   c. leukocytes.
   d. microbes.

6. Drugs that are effective against many pathogens are
   a. resistant.
   b. gram-stained.
   c. broad-spectrum.
   d. narrow-spectrum.

7. Pathogens are
   a. harmless microorganisms.
   b. infection-causing microorganisms.
   c. cancer cells.
   d. beneficial microbes.

8. An allergiclike reaction to a drug after taking several doses is
   a. resistance.
   b. sensitivity.
   c. superinfection.
   d. immunization.
9. Antimicrobial drugs fight infection by
   a. killing microorganisms directly.
   b. slowing the growth of microorganisms.
   c. stimulating the growth of microorganisms.
   d. both a and b.
10. Natural anti-infectives produced by one organism against another are
    a. antibiotics.
    b. sulfonamides.
    c. microorganisms.
    d. antiseptics.
11. A synthetic form of penicillin is
    a. amoxicillin.
    b. streptomycin.
    c. penicillin G.
    d. tetracycline.
12. A broad-spectrum antibiotic that should not be given with milk or antacids is
    a. amoxicillin (oral).
    b. chloramphenicol.
    c. gamma globulin.
    d. tetracycline.
13. A blood protein containing antibodies that protects the body from certain infections is
    a. neomycin.
    b. gamma globulin.
    c. sulfonamide.
    d. tetracycline.
14. Sulfonamides are most often used for
    a. headaches.
    b. respiratory infections.
    c. urinary infections.
    d. cancer treatment.
15. A patient has been on penicillin for 8 days. You notice that his tongue is taking on a black, furry appearance, which signals a mouth infection. This is an example of
    a. superinfection.
    b. resistance.
    c. hypersensitivity.
    d. penicillinase.

16. Which of the following is not a family of antibiotics?
    a. cephalosporins
    b. tetracyclines
    c. macrolides
    d. sulfonamides
17. Gram-staining and culture and sensitivity tests are ways to
    a. identify the germ causing a particular infection.
    b. find a drug that kills a particular pathogen.
    c. test a person's immunity.
    d. both a and b.
18. Airborne precautions are used in
    a. AIDS.
    b. tuberculosis.
    c. infected wound.
    d. scabies.
19. Reverse (protective) isolation is necessary in order to
    a. keep a patient from disturbing others.
    b. protect the patient from germs that medical staff are carrying.
    c. make medications work better.
    d. protect the medical staff from the patient's germs.
20. Contact precautions are used in
    a. chicken pox.
    b. mumps.
    c. herpes simplex.
    d. pertussis.
21. A severe, possibly fatal systemic hypersensitivity reaction to a drug is
    a. anaphylaxis.
    b. inoculation.
    c. vaccination.
    d. immunization.
22. A patient with tuberculosis should be placed in
    a. a four-bed unit.
    b. a two-bed room.
    c. a private room.
    d. the hallway.
23. Diseases caused by fungi are
    a. bacteriocidal.
    b. mycoses.
    c. superinfections.
    d. aseptic.
24. When giving medications to an isolation patient, it is important that you wash your hands
    a. before leaving the room.
    b. before entering the room.
    c. before and after giving medications.
    d. all of the above.

25. A broad-spectrum antibiotic is
    a. effective against a few pathogens.
    b. resistant to many pathogens.
    c. used when a narrow-spectrum antibiotic fails.
    d. capable of destroying a wide variety of microorganisms.
26. Antimicrobial drugs are discontinued
    a. as soon as the patient feels better.
    b. when diarrhea occurs.
    c. anytime the patient feels it is appropriate.
    d. when a patient is fever free for 48–72 hours.

Match the drug name(s) to the drug family.

______	27. penicillins	a. *Zovirax,* ganciclovir
______	28. cephalosporins	b. *Gantrisin,* sulfisoxazole, *Bactrim*
______	29. sulfonamides	c. *Fungizone, Nizoral,* miconazole
______	30. antivirals	d. ciprofloxacin, *Floxin, Noroxin*
______	31. antifungals	e. *Keflex, Keflin,* cephalexin
______	32. quinolones	f. EES, *Ilosone, Erythrocin*
______	33. macrolides	g. amikacin, gentamicin
______	34. aminoglycosides	h. *V-Cillin K, Pen-Vee K,* amoxicillin
______	35. erythromycins	i. *Achromycin-V, Vibramycin*

When you have passed this mastery test, sign up for a performance test on administering medications to an isolation patient.

Name ______________________ Date ______________________ Class ______________

Chapter 7 Test

Circle the letter of the best choice.

1. Diplopia is
   a. a bacterial infection of the eyelid.
   b. double vision.
   c. a hard cyst on the eyelid.
   d. increased pressure within the eye.
2. Tears are produced by the
   a. lacrimal gland.
   b. tragus.
   c. sclera.
   d. canthus.
3. The word that means pertaining to the ear is
   a. optic.
   b. olfactory.
   c. sensory.
   d. otic.
4. An alteration in the patient's perception of, or sensitivity to, sound is a
   a. conductive hearing loss.
   b. sensorineural hearing loss.
   c. central hearing loss.
   d. total deafness.
5. An eye disorder characterized by an increased intraocular pressure is
   a. conjunctivitis.
   b. blepharitis.
   c. glaucoma.
   d. hordeolum.
6. Cerumen is a greater problem in a(n)
   a. baby.
   b. child.
   c. adolescent.
   d. adult.
7. Hearing problems are caused by
   a. avoiding loud environmental noises.
   b. putting objects in the ears.
   c. getting all childhood immunizations.
   d. taking the full course of an antibiotic.
8. If an eyedrop lands on the outer eyelid when administering eyedrops,
   a. never administer another drop.
   b. ask the patient if he or she wants another drop.
   c. repeat administering the drop.
   d. take a cotton tip and push the drop in the eye.

9. When administering an eye ointment, instruct the patient to look
   a. up.
   b. down.
   c. straight ahead.
   d. sideways.
10. Drugs that dilate the pupil are
    a. carbonic anhydrase inhibitors.
    b. antibiotics.
    c. cycloplegias.
    d. mydriatics.
11. As a result of the aging process, the sclera becomes
    a. white.
    b. pink.
    c. red.
    d. yellow.
12. Ringing in the ears is
    a. cerumen.
    b. tinnitus.
    c. presbycusis.
    d. vertigo.
13. The transparent anterior portion of the eye is the
    a. lens.
    b. iris.
    c. sclera.
    d. cornea.
14. The part of the ear that stands out from the body is the
    a. auricle.
    b. eardrum.
    c. external auditory meatus.
    d. cerumen.
15. The membranes that line the eye sockets are the
    a. lacrimals.
    b. sclera.
    c. conjunctiva.
    d. humors.
16. A patient has a disorder of the eye that is being treated with pilocarpine. The disorder is probably
    a. glaucoma.
    b. tinnitus.
    c. presbyopia.
    d. conjunctivitis.

Place a T in the blank if the statement is true. Place an F in the blank if the statement is false.

______ 17. Drugs that expand the pupil are used to treat glaucoma.

______ 18. Because of the problem of blurring, eye ointments are often administered during the day and eyedrops at night.

______ 19. Because absorption through the conjunctiva is slow, eye medications must be very strong.

______ 20. Stinging and photophobia are side effects of some eye medications.

______ 21. A perforated eardrum must be treated like a mucous membrane.

______ 22. It is not necessary to clean the ear canal before instilling ear drops.

______ 23. To straighten the ear canal in a child, pull up and back on the top part of the ear.

______ 24. After instilling ear medication, ask the patient to stay in the same position for at least 5 minutes.

______ 25. For best effect, ear drops should be administered while they are cold.

After passing this mastery test, sign up for a performance test on

- instilling eyedrops and eye ointment.
- instilling ear drops.

Name ______________________ Date ______________________ Class ______________

Chapter 8 Test

Circle the letter of the best choice.

1. The function of the integumentary system is to
   a. protect the body from microorganisms.
   b. keep the body from drying out.
   c. insulate the body from cold.
   d. all of the above.
2. An antihistamine drug
   a. suppresses inflammation.
   b. relieves itching.
   c. works against the effects of histamines.
   d. kills parasites.
3. The signs of skin inflammation are swelling, warmth to the touch, pain, and
   a. redness.
   b. paleness.
   c. wrinkling.
   d. smoothness.
4. A person with dermatitis
   a. will be treated with a scabicide.
   b. has probably come in contact with an irritating substance.
   c. has a rash that itches.
   d. both b and c.
5. Which statement is true of psoriasis?
   a. It is easily cured.
   b. It causes red lesions with dry, silvery scales.
   c. It is treated with antibiotics.
   d. It is caused by an allergic reaction.
6. Normal body temperature is approximately
   a. 37° F.
   b. 96.8° F.
   c. 98.6° F.
   d. 96.8° C.
7. A patient complains of itching and hives. The doctor will probably order a(n)
   a. keratolytic.
   b. antibiotic.
   c. parasiticide.
   d. antipruritic.
8. Sweat is produced by the
   a. sebaceous glands.
   b. sudoriferous glands.
   c. ceruminous glands.
   d. subcutaneous tissue.

9. Greasy scales are a sign of
   a. acne.
   b. seborrheic dermatitis.
   c. dandruff.
   d. both b and c.

10. A thick, yellow fluid found in infected wounds is called
    a. pus.
    b. acne.
    c. cerumen.
    d. sebum.

11. Scabies and pediculosis are caused by
    a. fungi.
    b. insect stings.
    c. irritating cosmetics.
    d. mites and lice.

12. A drug like zinc oxide that forms a long-lasting film over a lesion so that it can heal better is called a(n)
    a. keratolytic.
    b. stimulant.
    c. antiseptic.
    d. protective.

13. Drugs that reduce swelling, reduce inflammation, and relieve itching are the
    a. corticosteroids.
    b. antibiotics.
    c. irritants.
    d. protectives.

14. Local anesthetics
    a. work by irritating the skin surface.
    b. suppress inflammation.
    c. relieve pain and itching.
    d. should not be used on sunburn.

15. A good way to ensure absorption into the skin layers is to
    a. keep the skin very dry.
    b. use a very weak concentration of the drug.
    c. apply an occlusive dressing if ordered.
    d. be careful not to rub the drug into the skin.

16. When there is a break in the skin and the underlying layers are exposed, use the same precautions as when medicating
    a. mucous membranes.
    b. unbroken skin.
    c. keratosis.
    d. the scalp.

17. Severe burns in which there is damage to the deeper tissue are treated
    a. with mild astringents and tonics.
    b. with keratolytics.
    c. under special instructions from a physician.
    d. with sunscreens.
18. While removing a patient's bandage, you find that it sticks to the wound. You should
    a. pull it off as gently as you can.
    b. soak it with sterile water and then pull it off gently.
    c. apply heat to soften the fibers.
    d. pull it off quickly to avoid hurting the patient.
19. Drugs that constrict the blood vessels and dry, weepy lesions are
    a. astringents.
    b. antibacterials.
    c. pediculicides.
    d. anesthetics.
20. Which of the following are examples of topical anti-inflammatory drugs (corticosteroids)?
    a. benzocaine, *Nupercanal*
    b. coal tar, menthol, salicylic acid
    c. neomycin, bacitracin, polymyxin B, *Sulfamylon*
    d. hydrocortisone, betametasone, *Aristocort, Cordran*

Match the medical terms in the left column with the appropriate description in the right column.

______	21. erythema	a. earwax
______	22. urticaria	b. hives
______	23. pruritus	c. itching
______	24. sebum	d. redness
______	25. cerumen	e. skin oil

When you have passed the mastery test, sign up for a performance test on applying topical medication to the skin.

Name ______________________ Date ____________________ Class ____________

Chapter 9 Test

Place a T in the blank if the statement is true. Place an F in the blank if the statement is false.

______ 1. An EKG is a device for measuring blood pressure.

______ 2. The exchange between oxygen and carbon dioxide takes place in the arteries.

______ 3. Blood is composed of plasma, red blood cells, white blood cells, and platelets.

______ 4. The average pulse is 60 to 80 beats per minute.

______ 5. Veins carry blood away from the heart.

______ 6. The vessels that nourish the heart are the coronary arteries.

Match the terms in the right column with the appropriate definition in the left column.

______	7. shortness of breath	a. angina
______	8. chest pain	b. dyspnea
______	9. swelling of tissues	c. hemorrhage
______	10. irregular heartbeat	d. arrhythmia
______	11. rapid heartbeat	e. tachycardia
______	12. bleeding	f. edema

Circle the letter of the best choice.

13. The lymphatic system is designed to
    a. filter the lymph.
    b. drain off excess fluid from spaces between cells.
    c. carry red blood cells to all parts of the body.
    d. a and b only.

14. The lymphatic system includes the lymph nodes and the
    a. heart.
    b. lungs.
    c. spleen.
    d. liver.

15. The average adult blood pressure is
    a. 120/80.
    b. 80/50.
    c. 180/90.
    d. 160/80.

16. Cyanosis is due to the lack of
    a. plasma in the blood.
    b. oxygen in the blood.
    c. nutrients in the blood.
    d. calcium in the blood.

17. Blood pressure increases as a result of
    a. narrowing of the blood vessels.
    b. widening of the blood vessels.
    c. thinning of the blood.
    d. thickening of the blood.
18. Patients with cardiovascular disease are usually placed on a
    a. low-sugar diet.
    b. low-salt diet.
    c. low-protein diet.
    d. low-carbohydrate diet.
19. Capillaries connect
    a. arteries to arteries.
    b. veins to veins.
    c. lymph vessels to arteries.
    d. arteries to veins.
20. Blood pressure is the result of the pumping action of the heart. It is
    a. the force exerted against the vessel walls.
    b. a feeling the heart is pounding or skipping beats.
    c. the force of the blood against the heart muscle.
    d. the force of the blood against lung tissue.
21. The technical term for high blood pressure is
    a. hypotension.
    b. hypertension.
    c. hypoglycemia.
    d. hyperthyroid.
22. Hemoglobin is found in the
    a. red blood cells.
    b. white blood cells.
    c. platelets.
    d. plasma.
23. A thrombus or air bubble that flows through the bloodstream is called
    a. an antibody.
    b. atherosclerosis.
    c. an embolus.
    d. phlebitis.
24. Collapse of the circulation due to injury, severe blood loss, surgery, or allergic reaction is called
    a. thrombophlebitis.
    b. leukemia.
    c. shock.
    d. congestive heart failure.

25. A condition in which the blood backs up from the heart into the veins and vital organs, causing swelling, is
    a. anemia.
    b. arrhythmia.
    c. varicose veins.
    d. congestive heart failure.
26. Atherosclerosis and arteriosclerosis
    a. are conditions that affect the blood vessels.
    b. can damage coronary arteries.
    c. may lead to angina or myocardial infarction.
    d. all of the above.
27. Lack of red blood cells and hemoglobin is called
    a. anemia.
    b. angina.
    c. Hodgkin's disease.
    d. hypotension.
28. The maintenance dose is
    a. the dose given regularly to keep up the level of a drug in the blood.
    b. the first few doses given in order to get the body adjusted to a drug.
    c. the last dose of a drug given before surgery.
    d. the amount of drug that can cause an overdose.
29. Antiarrhythmics
    a. act on the pacemaker cells that control the heartbeat.
    b. are heart depressants.
    c. reduce flutter and fibrillation.
    d. all of the above.
30. Drugs that stop blood clotting are
    a. antihypertensives.
    b. anticoagulants.
    c. antiarrhythmics.
    d. vasodilators.
31. Drugs like digitalis that increase the strength and force of the heart action are
    a. hemostatics.
    b. vasoconstrictors.
    c. vasodilators.
    d. heart stimulants.
32. Patients taking anticoagulants
    a. must have regular blood tests to adjust the dosage.
    b. must be observed for hemorrhage.
    c. are likely to be taking heparin, *Coumadin,* or dicumarol.
    d. all of the above.
33. Hematinics such as *Feosol* and *Imferon*
    a. provide iron for the red blood cells.
    b. are used to aid the clotting of blood.
    c. control hypertension.
    d. slow and steady the heartbeat.

34. Vitamin K (*Mephyton*) and thrombin are used topically as
    a. vasoconstrictors.
    b. vasodilators.
    c. diuretics.
    d. coagulants.
35. Nitroglycerin is a
    a. vasoconstrictor.
    b. vasodilator.
    c. diuretic.
    d. coagulant.
36. When giving a vasoconstrictor such as *Levophed* or *Intropin*,
    a. leave tablets by the bedside.
    b. weigh the patient daily.
    c. check blood pressure often.
    d. look for signs of digitalization.
37. When giving cardiovascular medications,
    a. read package inserts and drug references to become familiar with the drugs and their side effects.
    b. look for fatigue, dyspnea, or pain which may signal side effects.
    c. help the patient accept a new lifestyle.
    d. all of the above.
38. Take special care to dilute the preparation and administer it through a straw to avoid staining the teeth when giving
    a. antihypertensives.
    b. iron preparations.
    c. digitalis.
    d. heart depressants.
39. A patient was given 250 mg of *Aldomet*, an antihypertensive, this afternoon. This is the first time the patient received that medication, and the dosage will be adjusted according to the reaction. The patient feels faint when getting up to go to the bathroom. You are there right away to help because you have been watching for this sign of
    a. hypertension.
    b. hypotension.
    c. arrhythmia.
    d. hypertrophy.
40. A patient is to be given 0.25 mg of digoxin (*Lanoxin*) this morning. Digoxin is a digitalis product. Before administering his medication, you will
    a. take his blood pressure and chart it.
    b. read the EKG and chart it.
    c. give him a blood test.
    d. take his pulse and chart it.

When you have passed this mastery test, sign up for a performance test on

- administering oral medications.
- administering sublingual medications.

Name ______________________ Date ______________________ Class ______________

Chapter 10 Test

Match the part of the respiratory system in the right column to the appropriate function in the left column.

_____ 1. contains the vocal cords that make speech sounds

_____ 2. part of the muscle system that mechanically inflates the lungs

_____ 3. permit gases to be exchanged between the blood and the outside air

_____ 4. warm and moisten the air and trap dust and bacteria

_____ 5. pathway for both air and food

a. alveoli

b. diaphragm

c. pharynx

d. larynx

e. nasal cavities

Place a T in the blank if the statement is true. Place an F in the blank if the statement is false.

_____ 6. Percussion is the use of music therapy to relax respiratory patients.

_____ 7. A ventilating machine assists in the physical act of breathing.

_____ 8. The only effective treatment for respiratory problems is drug therapy.

_____ 9. A nebulizer creates a drug mist to be inhaled by the patient.

_____ 10. Respiratory patients can breathe better if they are lying flat on their backs.

_____ 11. Never give fluids with expectorants.

_____ 12. It is best not to trouble the patient's family by trying to explain respiration therapy.

_____ 13. Respiratory patients can get tired quickly when performing ordinary activities.

Circle the letter of the best choice.

14. Abnormal breathing sounds in the lungs can be heard using a
    a. cardiograph.
    b. sphygmomanometer.
    c. stethoscope.
    d. ventilator.
15. Normal respiratory rate is
    a. 12 to 25 times per minute.
    b. 10 to 15 times per minute.
    c. 20 to 27 times per minute.
    d. 30 to 40 times per minute.
16. Abnormally thick fluid that is formed in the lower respiratory tract and may be coughed up in bronchitis is
    a. mucous membrane.
    b. sputum.
    c. plasma.
    d. pus.

17. Which of the following is not a symptom of a respiratory problem?
    a. coughing
    b. hemoptysis
    c. iron lung
    d. nasal breathing
18. Which medical term would you use to describe a person who is breathing more rapidly and deeply than normal?
    a. dyspnea
    b. apnea
    c. hypernea
    d. tachycardia
19. A communicable or infectious disease that attacks the lung tissue is
    a. bronchitis.
    b. tuberculosis.
    c. emphysema.
    d. measles.
20. In viral bronchitis, the respiratory tract becomes plugged with thick mucus. It is therefore important to keep the air passages open and
    a. encourage fluids.
    b. discourage coughing.
    c. give antibiotics.
    d. avoid exercise.
21. A disorder in which the chest barrels out because the person cannot exhale properly is
    a. tuberculosis.
    b. emphysema.
    c. pleurisy.
    d. rhinitis.
22. Pneumonia is
    a. an allergy to pollen.
    b. a blood clot on the lung.
    c. an inflammation of the lining of the lungs.
    d. an infection of the lungs.
23. Rhinitis and sinusitis
    a. can be controlled with antibiotics if a bacteria can be identified.
    b. are inflammation of the nose and sinuses.
    c. have symptoms that can be controlled with decongestants and antihistamines.
    d. all of the above.
24. Bronchodilators such as epinephrine and aminophylline
    a. tighten the bronchioles.
    b. do not have any side effects.
    c. help asthma patients breathe more easily.
    d. are used to fight the common cold.

25. Which of the following methods are used to help the patient expectorate or to clear clogged passages?
    a. postural drainage
    b. percussion
    c. administration of antitussives
    d. all of the above
26. A patient has been in bed for a week recovering from lung surgery. While giving the routine medications, you notice that her nostrils are spreading slightly with each breath and she seems very tired. You should
    a. chart what you have seen and report it to your supervisor.
    b. forget it; it's probably a normal result of surgery.
    c. give her a sedative so she can get the rest she needs.
    d. give her nose drops for congestion.
27. Nose drops and nasal sprays
    a. carry medications deep into the lungs.
    b. are usually given for their systemic effects.
    c. treat only the area where they are applied.
    d. are administered by intermittent positive pressure breathing.
28. Respiratory therapists are specially trained to
    a. operate slipstream nebulizers and IPPB apparatus.
    b. administer inhalation therapy.
    c. write medication orders for respiratory drugs.
    d. a and b
29. Antitussives
    a. act on the cough center in the brain.
    b. stimulate a nonproductive cough.
    c. block the effects of histamine.
    d. kill the bacteria that cause pneumonia.
30. An example of a new, antihistamine is
    a. chlorpheniramine.
    b. acetaminophen.
    c. *Proventil.*
    d. *Zyrtec.*
31. Expectorants
    a. help the patient cough productively.
    b. shrink and dry the mucous membranes.
    c. thicken the sputum.
    d. relax the bronchioles.
32. Decongestants
    a. cure the underlying cause of congestion.
    b. thin and moisten mucous membranes.
    c. shrink and dry the mucous membranes.
    d. calm the urge to cough.

When you have passed this mastery test, sign up for a performance test on

- spraying medication onto mucous membranes of nose or throat.
- instilling nose drops or nasal sprays.

Name ______________________ Date ______________________ Class ______________

Chapter 11 Test

Circle the letter of the best choice.

1. The gastrointestinal system is designed to
   a. transport food along the alimentary canal.
   b. break down food into substances that can be absorbed.
   c. remove waste products from the body.
   d. all of the above.

2. An organ that secretes bile, removes waste products from the blood, and breaks down many drugs is the
   a. pancreas.
   b. liver.
   c. gallbladder.
   d. duodenum.

3. Intestinal motility is influenced by
   a. emotions.
   b. nervous system drugs.
   c. the presence of infections.
   d. all of the above.

4. A patient is having trouble with constipation because of a very inactive life. The doctor orders a laxative to be given as necessary. To help make the laxative more effective, you encourage the patient to
   a. take the laxative every day to prevent further constipation.
   b. avoid prunes and bran cereals.
   c. get more exercise.
   d. drink only one glass of water per day.

5. How are constipation, nausea, and ulcers affected by nervous tension?
   a. Nervous tension makes them worse.
   b. Nervous tension makes them better.
   c. Nervous tension has no effect one way or another.
   d. Nervous tension makes some disorders better and some worse.

6. Gastrointestinal medications are affected by whether there is food in the stomach. Therefore, they should
   a. be given before, after, during, or between mealtimes as ordered.
   b. always be given before meals.
   c. always be given between meals.
   d. always be given with food.

7. After you have inserted a rectal suppository, watch for signs of
   a. fatigue and fever.
   b. pain and irritation in the rectal area.
   c. bowel movements that occur right after insertion.
   d. b and c.

8. When you insert a rectal suppository
   a. do not wear a glove.
   b. press the buttocks together until the urge to defecate passes.
   c. keep the wrapper on during insertion to prevent contamination.
   d. dissolve the suppository before insertion.
9. Emetics like syrup of ipecac are used
   a. to produce vomiting.
   b. to prevent motion sickness.
   c. to relieve nausea.
   d. to slow peristalsis.
10. Antihistamines and tranquilizers that are used to control nausea and vomiting are called
    a. antispasmodics.
    b. anticholinergics.
    c. antiemetics.
    d. cathartics.
11. Anticholinergics slow intestinal motility by acting on the autonomic nervous system. They also
    a. slow the production of stomach acid.
    b. can cause blurred vision, dilated pupils, constipation, and inability to urinate.
    c. block the action of acetylcholine.
    d. all of the above.
12. Drugs that slow intestinal motility or have an astringent, absorbent, and demulcent action on the intestines are called
    a. antidiarrheals.
    b. laxatives.
    c. anorexiants.
    d. antihelmintics.
13. Drugs that stimulate the large intestine, increase bulk, soften stools, and hold water in the large intestine are called
    a. antidiarrheals.
    b. cathartics.
    c. anticholinergics.
    d. antiemetics.
14. A sore or a break in the lining of the stomach or duodenum caused by excess stomach acid is called a(n)
    a. stoma.
    b. hemorrhoid.
    c. polyp.
    d. ulcer.
15. Intestinal parasites such as pinworms and roundworms are treated with
    a. antihelmintics.
    b. antiflatulents.
    c. antacids.
    d. anorexiants.

16. Jaundice, hepatitis, and cirrhosis are disorders of the
    a. pancreas.
    b. gallbladder.
    c. liver.
    d. small intestine.
17. Calcium carbonate, aluminum hydroxide, and magnesium hydroxide
    a. are called antacids.
    b. neutralize stomach acid.
    c. are used in the treatment of ulcers.
    d. all of the above.
18. Drugs that replace the enzymes that break down fat, protein, and sugar are called
    a. diuretics.
    b. digestants.
    c. anticholinergics.
    d. purgatives.
19. Antiflatulents or carminatives are added to antacid preparations to
    a. aid the passing of gas.
    b. stimulate gastric secretions.
    c. provide a sedative effect.
    d. cause vomiting.
20. Reversal of peristalsis is called
    a. emesis.
    b. diarrhea.
    c. constipation.
    d. defecation.
21. A tube that is used to feed and administer drugs through the nose and esophagus is called a(n)
    a. gastrostomy tube.
    b. proctoscope.
    c. nasogastric tube.
    d. sigmoidoscope.
22. When inserting a rectal suppository, be sure to place it
    a. beyond the anal rectal ridge.
    b. beyond the epiglottis.
    c. into the feces.
    d. at least 8 inches into the rectum.
23. Absorption of nutrients from the gastrointestinal tract takes place mainly in the
    a. stomach.
    b. liver.
    c. large intestine.
    d. small intestine.

24. As you give a patient medications, the patient complains of abdominal pain. This is the first time the patient, who has been under your care for several days, has mentioned this symptom. You should
    a. chart and mention this symptom to the physician or the nurse in charge.
    b. give the patient a laxative, since he probably has constipation.
    c. withhold food for several days.
    d. do not do anything, just wait and see if he feels better in a few hours.
25. When giving medications through a nasogastric or gastrostomy tube,
    a. crush timed release medications.
    b. mix all medications together before giving.
    c. give one medication at a time.
    d. mix medications with normal saline.
26. You are giving a patient medications through a gastrostomy tube when you notice the stoma is leaking and showing redness and pus around the edges. You should
    a. patch the leak with band aids.
    b. hold off giving the medications until the next day.
    c. notify your supervisor immediately.
    d. apply a topical anti-infective.
27. Which of the following does not have an anticholinergic or antispasmodic action?
    a. atropine sulfate with phenobarbital (*Donnatal*)
    b. propantheline bromide (*Pro-Banthine*)
    c. milk of magnesia
    d. dicyclomine (*Bentyl*)
28. Examples of antiemetics are
    a. prochlorperazine (*Compazine*) and meclizine (*Antivert*).
    b. belladonna and atropine sulfate.
    c. kaolin and pectin.
    d. thiabendazole (*Mintezol*) and quinarcrin (*Atabrine*).
29. Which of the following medications is a Histamine H_2-Receptor Antagonist?
    a. Docusate sodium (Colace)
    b. Prochlorperazine (Compazine)
    c. Meclizine (Antivert)
    d. Iansoprazole (Prevacid)

After you have passed this mastery test, sign up for a performance test on

- inserting a rectal suppository.
- administering medication through an installed nasogastric or gastrostomy tube.

Name ______________________ Date ______________________ Class ______________

Chapter 12 Test

Circle the letter of the best choice.

1. The urinary system carries out its functions by filtering the blood. This process takes place in the
   a. ureters.
   b. kidneys.
   c. bladder.
   d. urethra.
2. Before being eliminated from the body, urine is stored in the
   a. kidneys.
   b. ureters.
   c. bladder.
   d. urethra.
3. The balance of acids to alkalis (bases) is called
   a. pH balance.
   b. fluid balance.
   c. acidosis.
   d. acid balance.
4. After the blood is filtered in the glomeruli
   a. all the liquids and salts are eliminated from the body.
   b. all the liquids and salts are reabsorbed in the nephrons.
   c. some of the liquids and salts are reabsorbed and some are eliminated.
   d. the red blood cells pass out of the body.
5. Dysuria, oliguria, anuria, and incontinence
   a. are revealed by urine tests.
   b. are difficulties with urination.
   c. may be side effects of drugs that affect the nervous system.
   d. both b and c.
6. Blood and pus in the urine
   a. are revealed by urine tests.
   b. may be signs of disorders in the kidney.
   c. are known as hematuria and pyuria.
   d. all of the above.
7. A plastic tube inserted into the bladder to permit drainage of urine is called a
   a. cystoscope.
   b. catheter.
   c. urinometer.
   d. dialysis machine.
8. All of the following are urinary system disorders except
   a. kidney failure.
   b. urethritis.
   c. nephritis.
   d. neuritis.

9. People who administer medications should understand kidney functions and disorders because
   a. the kidneys are involved in excretion of drugs.
   b. kidneys that do not work properly can lead to cumulation of drugs.
   c. antibiotics can be damaging to the kidneys.
   d. all of the above.

10. When the body excretes more water than it takes in, the result is
    a. edema.
    b. dehydration.
    c. pH imbalance.
    d. uremia.

11. Examples of fluid output that should be charted are
    a. drinks of water or juice.
    b. IV infusions.
    c. vomited liquids.
    d. tube-fed liquids.

12. A lack of potassium is called
    a. hypokalemia.
    b. hypocalcemia.
    c. hyponatremia.
    d. hypochondria.

13. Electrolytes
    a. are dissolved mineral salts.
    b. are involved in chemical exchanges in the body fluids.
    c. are not really necessary for proper body functioning.
    d. a and b.

14. Acidifiers such as vitamin C, ammonium chloride, and cranberry juice
    a. make the body's pH more alkaline.
    b. may be given to help certain drugs have their strongest effect.
    c. may be given to counteract alkalosis.
    d. both b and c.

15. Urinary antiseptics
    a. become active when they are excreted by the kidneys.
    b. are sometimes combined with analgesics.
    c. may be given by catheter.
    d. all of the above.

16. Drugs that decrease the reabsorption of water and salts from the nephrons are called
    a. dehydrators.
    b. urinary antiseptics.
    c. diuretics.
    d. alkalizers.

17. A bladder infection involving painful spasms and frequent urination is
    a. pyelonephritis.
    b. edema.
    c. dehydration.
    d. cystitis.

18. Nalidixic acid (*Neg Gram*) and nitrofurantoin (*Macrodantin*) are examples of
    a. urinary analgesics.
    b. urinary antiseptics.
    c. diuretics.
    d. electrolyte replacements.

19. A danger with diuretics is
    a. over- or underexcretion of potassium.
    b. orthostatic hypotension.
    c. electrolyte imbalances.
    d. all of the above.

20. *Slow-K,* Ringer's solution, and *Kaon* are examples of
    a. diuretics.
    b. replacement electrolytes and fluids.
    c. urinary antiseptics.
    d. urinary analgesics.

21. You are giving a patient a diuretic to control edema. You take care to give the drug at the correct time of day, and you make sure that the call button is within the patient's reach. This is because the patient will
    a. urinate more frequently.
    b. have a big appetite.
    c. stay awake at night.
    d. have increased pitting of the skin.

22. *Pedialyte, Lytren,* and *Resol* are examples of
    a. urinary antiseptics.
    b. diuretics.
    c. urinary analgesics.
    d. oral replacement solutions.

23. Rinsing the bladder with sterile water and/or an anti-infective is called
    a. bladder irrigation.
    b. bladder intubation.
    c. bladder retention.
    d. bladder gavage.

24. When instilling medication through a urinary catheter,
    a. make sure the liquid is the right temperature.
    b. use aseptic procedure to avoid contamination.
    c. hook up or unclamp the drainage tube after the prescribed amount of time.
    d. all of the above.

25. Chlorothiazide (*Diuril*) and hydrochlorothiazide (*HydroDIURIL*) are
    a. potassium-sparing diuretics.
    b. thiazide diuretics.
    c. osmotic diuretics.
    d. mercurial diuretics.
26. Children are very susceptible to the effects of diuretics because of
    a. a large percentage of body fat.
    b. overdeveloped kidneys.
    c. a larger percentage of body water.
    d. thick and impermeable skin.
27. To prevent urinary tract infections, women should
    a. use vaginal sprays daily.
    b. wipe from back to front after having a bowel movement.
    c. wear synthetic underwear.
    d. take showers instead of baths.

After you have passed this mastery test, sign up for a performance test on instilling medication into the bladder through an indwelling catheter.

Name ______________________ Date ______________________ Class ______________

Chapter 13 Test

Circle the letter of the best choice.

1. Female sex cells are produced by the
   a. ovaries.
   b. uterus.
   c. testes.
   d. vagina.
2. The structure that holds the fertilized ovum while it develops inside the woman's body is the
   a. ovary.
   b. uterus.
   c. perineum.
   d. vagina.
3. The vulva, mons pubis, and labia are parts of the
   a. female internal genitalia.
   b. female external genitalia.
   c. male internal genitalia.
   d. male external genitalia.
4. Methyltestosterone (*Android*) and testosterone propionate (*Oreton*) are
   a. male hormones.
   b. female hormones.
   c. contraceptives.
   d. muscle relaxants.
5. The male external genitalia consist of
   a. the penis and the scrotum.
   b. the testes and the epididymis.
   c. the prostate gland and the vas deferens.
   d. the seminal vesicles.
6. Another term for male and female sex glands is
   a. gonads.
   b. gonadotrophins.
   c. ova.
   d. spermatozoa.
7. The pituitary gland secretes LH and FSH, which help regulate the ovaries and the testes. The pituitary hormones are known as
   a. gonads.
   b. gonadotrophins.
   c. menses.
   d. oxytocins.
8. A hormone that stimulates the production of milk by the mammary glands is
   a. progesterone.
   b. estrogen.
   c. prolactin.
   d. oxytocin.

9. The pituitary gland secretes oxytocin to
   a. cause uterine contractions.
   b. stimulate ovulation.
   c. stimulate the testes to produce testosterone.
   d. all of the above.

10. Vaginitis and cervicitis may be treated with
    a. topical douches, creams, tablets, and suppositories.
    b. vaginal antibacterials.
    c. *Monistat 7*, *Gyne-Lotrimin*, AVC cream, *Sultrin*.
    d. all of the above.

11. The hormone responsible for female shapeliness, higher voice, and the development of ova is
    a. progesterone.
    b. estrogen.
    c. prolactin.
    d. oxytocin.

12. Syphilis and gonorrhea
    a. are sexually transmitted diseases.
    b. are spread by sexual contact.
    c. are treated with penicillin and other antibiotics.
    d. all of the above.

13. It is very common for men 40 to 70 years of age to develop infections or cancer in the
    a. bladder.
    b. prostate.
    c. testes.
    d. Cowper's glands.

14. The hormone that stimulates sperm production and the development of a deep voice, chest hair, and facial hair is
    a. progesterone.
    b. dydrogesterone.
    c. testosterone.
    d. estrone.

15. A patient is suffering from dysmenorrhea, so the physican prescribes small doses of estrogen. Dysmenorrhea is
    a. labor contractions.
    b. ovulation.
    c. painful menstruation.
    d. breast engorgement.

16. Estradiol and estrone are forms of
    a. estrogen.
    b. progesterone.
    c. testosterone.
    d. androgens.

17. The hormone that prepares the uterus to nourish a growing fetus is
    a. progesterone.
    b. estrogen.
    c. prolactin.
    d. oxytocin.

18. All of the following are uses of sex hormones except
    a. relieving the symptoms of menopause.
    b. controlling certain forms of cancer.
    c. replacing missing hormones.
    d. stimulating the development of osteoporosis.

19. The drug of choice in the treatment of trichomoniasis is
    a. metronidazole (*Flagyl*).
    b. danazol (*Danocrine*).
    c. acyclovir (*Zovirax*).
    d. terazosin (*Hytrin*).

20. The female gonads secrete
    a. estrogen.
    b. progesterone.
    c. testosterone.
    d. a and b.

21. Trichomoniasis is a common infection of women involving the
    a. bladder.
    b. vagina.
    c. Fallopian tubes.
    d. uterus.

22. Chlamydial infection, a sexually transmitted disease, is common and can have serious complications including
    a. infertility.
    b. blindness.
    c. pelvic inflammatory disease.
    d. a and c only.

23. Drugs used to treat infertility problems include
    a. clomiphene and menotropins.
    b. estrogen and progesterone.
    c. estrogen and estrone.
    b. acyclovir and *Flagyl*.

24. The drug given to relieve hot flashes and other discomforts of menopause is
    a. testosterone.
    b. metronidazole.
    c. estrogen.
    d. progesterone.

25. In addition to their role in reproduction, sex hormones are involved with
    a. growth and bone formation.
    b. storage of minerals.
    c. building proteins.
    d. all of the above.

After you have passed this mastery test, sign up for a performance test on inserting vaginal medication.

Name ______________________ Date ____________________ Class ____________

Chapter 14 Test

Circle the letter of the best choice.

1. Glands combine chemicals to produce
   a. globulins.
   b. hormones.
   c. somatotropes.
   d. parathyroids.

2. Corticosteroids such as prednisone and dexamethasone are most often used because of their
   a. anti-inflammatory action.
   b. sedative action.
   c. anti-infective action.
   d. diuretic action.

3. Diabetics take blood tests to determine the presence of
   a. sugar and ketones.
   b. water and sodium.
   c. protein.
   d. potassium.

4. The islets of Langerhans, which secrete insulin and glucagon, are located in the
   a. thyroid.
   b. pancreas.
   c. liver.
   d. adrenals.

5. The newest long-acting insulin available that eliminates the need for multiple daily injections is
   a. *Ultralente.*
   b. glyburide.
   c. *Humulin N.*
   d. Humalog.

6. The medical term for sugar in the urine is
   a. tetany.
   b. glycosuria.
   c. polyuria.
   d. hypoglycemia.

7. Diabetes insipidus is caused by a lack of
   a. antidiuretic hormone.
   b. insulin.
   c. glucocorticoids.
   d. mineralocorticoids.

8. Regular and semilente are
    a. fast-acting insulins.
    b. intermediate-acting insulins.
    c. long-lasting insulins.
    d. oral hypoglycemics.
9. Cortisone and hydrocortisone are natural
    a. insulins.
    b. anticholesteremics.
    c. corticosteroids.
    d. testosterones.
10. The gland that traps iodine to produce thyroxine is called the
    a. pancreas.
    b. parathyroid.
    c. thyroid.
    d. pituitary.
11. Somatotropic hormone, antidiuretic hormone, and many hormones that regulate other glands are secreted by the
    a. pancreas.
    b. ovaries.
    c. parathyroids.
    d. pituitary.
12. Parathormone regulates
    a. the use of sugar by the cells.
    b. the level of calcium in the bloodstream.
    c. the reaction of the body to stress.
    d. the secretions of the adrenal cortex.
13. Tolbuamide (*Orinase*) and chlorpropamide (*Diabinese*) are
    a. fast-acting insulins.
    b. intermediate-acting insulins.
    c. long-lasting insulins.
    d. oral hypoglycemics.
14. Thyroxine regulates
    a. the speed at which the body burns nutrients for heat and energy.
    b. the production of corticosteroids by the adrenals.
    c. the reabsorption of water in the kidneys.
    d. the release of stored sugar into the bloodstream from the liver.
15. A disease caused by lack of insulin is
    a. diabetes insipidus.
    b. diabetes mellitus.
    c. hypoglycemia.
    d. aldosteronism.
16. Corticotropin (ACTH) may be administered to
    a. stimulate the adrenals.
    b. diagnose pituitary disorders.
    c. stimulate growth.
    d. both a and b.

17. In a diabetic patient, extreme hunger, sweating, confusion, palpitations, and restlessness during sleep may be signs of
    a. hypoglycemia.
    b. insulin underdose.
    c. diabetic coma.
    d. glycosuria.
18. Drugs used in the treatment of hypothyroidism are
    a. *Diabinese, Orinase, Tolinase.*
    b. methylprednisolone, prednisone, *Decadron.*
    c. Glucagon, Regular and NPH insulin
    d. *Synthroid, Cytomel, Thyrolar.*
19. Hypertension, "moon" face, edema, thinning skin, and salt retention are important side effects of
    a. corticosteroids.
    b. insulin.
    c. oral hypoglycemics.
    d. parathormone.
20. Excessive thirst, production of excess urine, weakness, and glycosuria are symptoms of
    a. insulin shock.
    b. lack of insulin.
    c. insulin overdose.
    d. hypoglycemia.
21. Corticosteroids are ordered with care because
    a. they may mask infection.
    b. they have dangerous side effects in long-term use.
    c. they may interfere with the hormone control system between the adrenals and the pituitary.
    d. all of the above.
22. Which of the following conditions may require an adjustment in the diabetic's dosage of insulin?
    a. emotional stress and other drugs
    b. heavy exercise
    c. a change in diet
    d. all of the above
23. The presence of many fatty acids in the bloodstream of a diabetic person leads to an imbalance in the body's pH. This condition is called
    a. ketoalkalosis.
    b. ketoacidosis.
    c. hypothyroid.
    d. glycosuria.
24. Addison's disease, a long-term malfunction of the adrenals, is treated by replacement of
    a. corticosteroids.
    b. insulin.
    c. parathormone.
    d. antidiuretic hormone.

25. You have just given a patient an injection of regular insulin. You know that its action peaks in about 2 or 3 hours. It is important for you to know this so that you can
    a. put the patient to bed at that time.
    b. withhold snacks at that time.
    c. be alert for signs of hypoglycemia at that time.
    d. give the next dose of insulin.
26. Insulin suspensions
    a. should be shaken vigorously before administration.
    b. should be discarded if they contain clumps and granules.
    c. should be rotated gently between the palms and tipped end to end before administration.
    d. both b and c.
27. In case of insulin shock, give
    a. two glasses of water.
    b. coffee or tea.
    c. orange juice or candy.
    d. extra insulin.
28. *Humulin N* is
    a. fast acting.
    b. intermediate acting.
    c. long acting.
    d. both a and b.
29. *Humulin R* is
    a. fast acting.
    b. intermediate acting.
    c. long acting.
    d. both a and b.
30. Oral hypoglycemic agents are most effective in a patient
    a. less than 40 years of age.
    b. who has been diabetic less than 5 years.
    c. who has a fluctuating diet.
    d. who has been controlled on 80 units of insulin daily.

Name ______________________ Date ______________________ Class ______________

Chapter 15 Test

Circle the letter of the best choice.

1. Tendons
   a. connect muscles to bones.
   b. connect bones together at the joints.
   c. are membranes that cover the muscles.
   d. all of the above.
2. The red bone marrow manufactures all of the following except
   a. red blood cells.
   b. certain white blood cells.
   c. uric acid crystals.
   d. platelets.
3. A sign that an arthritis patient has taken too much aspirin is
   a. ringing in the ears.
   b. increased joint pain.
   c. severe itching.
   d. all of the above.
4. The main side effect of antiarthritics is that you should be alert for
   a. blurred vision.
   b. gastrointestinal upset.
   c. fever.
   d. itching.
5. Because patients with musculoskeletal conditions are often in pain, be sure to
   a. have them exercise the joints before taking medications.
   b. give medications for pain only several hours after the last dose has worn off.
   c. ignore their fears and psychological needs so that they do not dwell on them.
   d. avoid sudden, jarring movements, and support body parts if they must be moved.
6. All the following are used to relieve the symptoms of rheumatoid arthritis except
   a. colchicine, allopurinol, *Colbenemid.*
   b. aspirin, *Ecotrin.*
   c. indomethacin (*Indocin*), ibuprofen (*Motrin*), sulindac (*Clinoril*).
   d. gold compounds.
7. Methocarbamol (*Robaxin*), *Parafon Forte,* cyclobenzaprine (*Flexeril*), and tubocurarine are types of
   a. muscle relaxants.
   b. analgesics.
   c. corticosteroids.
   d. anti-inflammatory drugs.

8. Gold compounds and antimalarial drugs are sometimes used in the treatment of
   a. gout.
   b. rheumatoid arthritis.
   c. muscle pain.
   d. prostatitis.
9. An inflammation of the synovial capsule that destroys the cartilage in the joints and causes pain, stiffness, warmth, and sometimes crippling is called
   a. rheumatoid arthritis.
   b. gouty arthritis.
   c. arthroplasty.
   d. osteoarthritis.
10. Bursitis, fibrositis, and synovitis
    a. are inflammations of the joints.
    b. may be treated with injections of hydrocortisone and oral anti-inflammatory drugs.
    c. are infections of the bone.
    d. both a and b.
11. Muscle relaxants are used to
    a. relieve pain of arthritis and orthopedic conditions.
    b. relieve overuse injuries of the muscles.
    c. prepare patients for certain types of surgery and for electroshock therapy.
    d. all of the above.
12. Bones are hard because they contain deposits of
    a. calcium.
    b. bone marrow.
    c. fat.
    d. iodine.
13. A buildup of uric acid crystals in the joints is called
    a. gout.
    b. rheumatoid arthritis.
    c. osteomyelitis.
    d. tendonitis.
14. Muscles that move the large bones of the body are called
    a. fascia.
    b. cardiac muscles.
    c. smooth muscles.
    d. skeletal muscles.
15. Joint pain and stiffness caused by wear and tear from bones rubbing together is known as
    a. rheumatoid arthritis.
    b. gouty arthritis.
    c. osteoarthritis.
    d. osteoporosis.

16. Uricosurics and antihyperuricemics
    a. prevent or reduce the formation of uric acid crystals in the joints.
    b. promote the buildup of uric acid in the bloodstream.
    c. cause the production of large amounts of uric acid.
    d. are types of corticosteroids.
17. Oral corticosteroids are sometimes given to reduce inflammation in rheumatoid arthritis. What side effect limits their usefulness?
    a. bone thinning
    b. peptic ulcers
    c. psychological changes
    d. all of the above
18. Pain in the skeletal muscles is known as
    a. tendonitis.
    b. rheumatoid arthritis.
    c. myalgia.
    d. osteomyelitis.
19. The antimalarial drug chloroquine is sometimes given to relieve the symptoms of
    a. myalgia.
    b. rheumatoid arthritis.
    c. bursitis.
    d. gout.
20. All of the following drugs are used to treat gout except
    a. sulfinpyrazone.
    b. *Colbenemid.*
    c. *Zyloprim.*
    d. aspirin.
21. An example of a synarthrotic joint is the
    a. skull.
    b. hip.
    c. pelvis.
    d. ankle.
22. A new revolutionary drug used to treat osteoarthritis is
    a. aspirin.
    b. *Fosamax.*
    c. rofecoxila.
    d. metotrexate.

Name ____________________ Date ____________________ Class ____________

Chapter 16 Test

Circle the letter of the best choice.

1. The central nervous system consists of the
   a. nerves and sense receptors.
   b. brain and spinal cord.
   c. cerebrum and cerebellum.
   d. nerves and spinal cord.
2. The autonomic nervous system
   a. regulates the internal organs automatically.
   b. gears the body up for fighting stress.
   c. restores body functions to normal after danger is past.
   d. all of the above.
3. Neurons have long branches that are responsible for
   a. transmitting nerve impulses.
   b. linking the CNS to all parts of the body.
   c. sending information collected by the sense receptors.
   d. all of the above.
4. A patient is showing signs of tremor and bradykinesia. This means he is
   a. shaking and moving very slowly.
   b. in a daze.
   c. paralyzed.
   d. overly excited.
5. The medical term for dizziness is
   a. stupor.
   b. psychosis.
   c. coma.
   d. vertigo.
6. Shaking, stiffness, and slowness of movement are the classic symptoms of
   a. Meniere's disease.
   b. Parkinson's disease.
   c. epilepsy.
   d. brain tumor.
7. The disorder involving periodic seizures or convulsions is called
   a. diplopia.
   b. Parkinson's disease.
   c. epilepsy.
   d. multiple sclerosis.
8. A cerebrovascular accident or stroke is
   a. a disorder of the ear.
   b. a hemorrhage or blood clot on the brain.
   c. a sign of psychosis.
   d. a nerve disease.

9. Inflammations that affect the CNS are
   a. conjunctivitis, sty.
   b. otitis, Meniere's disease.
   c. meningitis, encephalitis.
   d. neuritis, neuralgia.
10. Drugs that make the nervous system work faster, such as amphetamines, are called
    a. stimulants.
    b. depressants.
    c. receptors.
    d. barbiturates.
11. Examples of antiparkinsonian drugs are
    a. *Demerol*, *Percodan*, and *Talwin*.
    b. *Nuprin*, *Motrin*, and *Tylenol* with Codeine.
    c. *Dilantin* and phenobarbital.
    d. *Levodopa*, *Symmetrel*, and *Sinemet*.
12. Examples of CNS depressants are
    a. tranquilizers and antipsychotic drugs.
    b. pain relievers and sedatives.
    c. anticonvulsants and anesthetics.
    d. all of the above.
13. Analgesic antipyretics relieve pain and
    a. kill microorganisms.
    b. stimulate the nervous system.
    c. reduce fever.
    d. all of the above.
14. Along with pain relief, narcotic analgesics
    a. bring euphoria and a sense of calm.
    b. reduce inflammation.
    c. can cause physical dependence.
    d. a and c.
15. Morphine, propoxyphene (*Darvon*), and meperidine (*Demerol*) are
    a. amphetamines.
    b. analgesics.
    c. ophthalmic preparations.
    d. anticonvulsants.
16. Pentobarbital (*Nembutal*) and phenobarbital are examples of
    a. antipsychotics.
    b. amphetamines.
    c. barbiturates.
    d. narcotics.
17. *Dilantin*, *Depakote*, and *Tegretol* are
    a. antianxiety agents.
    b. antipsychotics.
    c. sedatives.
    d. anticonvulsants.

18. Always give analgesics
    a. after the last dose has worn off.
    b. just before the last dose has worn off.
    c. only when the patient seems to be in pain.
    d. at bedtime.
19. Dryness of the mouth (a side effect of some CNS stimulants) can be relieved by
    a. hard candy.
    b. sugarless gum.
    c. rinsing the mouth with water.
    d. all of the above.

Name ______________________ Date ______________________ Class ______________

Chapter 17 Test

Circle the letter of the best choice.

1. Examples of antidepressant drugs are
   a. *Haldol, Prolixin,* and *Stelazine.*
   b. parnate, *Tofranil,* and *Zoloft.*
   c. *Valium, Dalmane,* and *Serax.*
   d. *Benadryl, Cogentin,* and *Restoril.*

2. Examples of CNS depressants are
   a. tranquilizers and antipsychotic drugs.
   b. pain relievers and sedatives.
   c. anticonvulsants and anesthetics.
   d. all of the above.

3. *Valium, Librium, Serax,* and *Atarax* are
   a. antianxiety drugs.
   b. antipsychotic drugs.
   c. sedatives.
   d. antimanic agents.

4. Antipsychotics such as chlorpromazine (*Thorazine*) and thioridazine (*Melleril*)
   a. are minor tranquilizers.
   b. are used in the treatment of manic-depressive illness.
   c. may cause extrapyramidal symptoms.
   d. are rendered ineffective if taken with alcohol.

5. Drugs used to treat the manic episode of a manic depressive illness are
   a. sedatives.
   b. minor tranquilizers.
   c. barbiturates.
   d. antimanics.

6. A state of psychologically induced immobilization at times interrupted by episodes of extreme agitation is
   a. dystonia.
   b. catatonia.
   c. insomnia.
   d. mania.

7. Irreversible repetitious movements of the face, limbs, and trunk after an antipsychotic drug is
   a. tardive dyskinesia.
   b. a delusion.
   c. akathisia.
   d. dystonia.

8. Psychosis is a classic feature in
   a. anxiety.
   b. sedation.
   c. schizophrenia.
   d. depression.

9. Anxiety is
   a. an inability to recognize reality.
   b. a physiological and psychological mechanism protecting an individual from a threatening situation.
   c. a false belief that is resistant to reasoning.
   d. a sense of worthlessness resulting in the inability to carry out normal activities.

10. Diazepam (*Valium*), lorazepam (*Ativan*), and oxazepam (*Serax*) are examples of
    a. antipsychotics.
    b. antimanic drugs.
    c. antianxiety drugs.
    d. antidepressants.

11. Patients taking lithium should be taught to
    a. limit their daily fluid intake to 1000 ml.
    b. exercise routinely.
    c. increase their weight.
    d. avoid coffee, tea, and cola.

12. The most common side effects of lithium are
    a. tremors of the hands, thirst, nausea, increased urination, and diarrhea.
    b. orthostatic hypotension, blurred vision, sedation, and constipation.
    c. involuntary movements around the mouth, lips, and tongue.
    d. agitation, increased strength, elevated temperature, and weight loss.

13. Minor tranquilizers are also
    a. antipsychotics.
    b. antidepressants.
    c. antimanic drugs.
    d. antianxiety drugs.

14. Examples of monoamine oxidase (MAO) inhibitors are
    a. *Nardil, Marplan,* and *Parnate.*
    b. *Pamelor, Tofranil,* and *Ascendin.*
    c. *Effexor, Anafranil,* and *Ludiomil.*
    d. *Zoloft, Prozac,* and *Wellbutrin.*

15. A patient is sedated following a serious accident. You can enhance the effect of the sedation by
    a. turning up the volume on the television set.
    b. letting the patient take frequent naps during the day.
    c. avoiding any talk about the patient's fears and worries.
    d. giving the patient a back rub or a warm bath.

16. The best time to give p.r.n. sedatives is when
    a. the patient is in pain.
    b. you are tired of listening to the patient's complaints.
    c. the patient still needs them after you have done everything else to relax the patient.
    d. the vital signs show the nervous system is overdepressed.
17. *Thorazine, Stelazine,* and *Prolixin* are
    a. antianxiety drugs.
    b. antipsychotics.
    c. antimanics.
    d. antidepressants.
18. Caution should be used when giving psychiatric drugs to
    a. alcoholics.
    b. overweight individuals.
    c. diabetics.
    d. individuals with arthritis.
19. Examples of hallucinogens are
    a. morphine and *Demerol.*
    b. alcohol and seconal.
    c. methadone and opium.
    d. LSD and marijuana.
20. Drugs in the sedative/hypnotic category include
    a. *Atarax* and *Dalmane.*
    b. *Trilafon* and *Serentil.*
    c. *Demerol* and morphine.
    d. *Cogentin* and *Benadryl.*
21. Two drugs used to treat an attention deficit hyperactivity disorder (ADHD) in a pediatric patient are
    a. lorazepam and *Restoril.*
    b. *Adderall* and methylphenidate.
    c. imipramine and *Elavil.*
    d. *Prozac* and fluphenazine.

Name ______________________ Date ______________________ Class ______________

Chapter 18 Test

Circle the letter of the best choice.

1. The smallest living units in the human body are
   a. cells.
   b. systems.
   c. tissues.
   d. organs.
2. The ability of the body to replace damaged cells is
   a. reproduction.
   b. healing.
   c. cytoplasm.
   d. specialization.
3. The fluid found inside the cells is
   a. cytoplasm.
   b. tissue fluid.
   c. edema.
   d. gamma globulin.
4. Chemotherapy works by
   a. searching out and killing only cancer cells.
   b. destroying rapidly growing cells, including cancer cells.
   c. stimulating the body's defense system.
   d. making the body immune to cancer.
5. Assist chemotherapy patients by
   a. helping with oral hygiene and nutrition.
   b. following aseptic procedure to prevent infection.
   c. charting new infections and signs of stomach or intestinal distress.
   d. all of the above.
6. Cancer cells are known to
   a. grow and divide more rapidly than normal cells.
   b. invade nearby healthy tissues.
   c. metastasize to other parts of the body.
   d. all of the above.
7. Antineoplastics are drugs that
   a. nourish cancer cells.
   b. protect the body from infection.
   c. stop the growth of tumors.
   d. cause tumors to grow.
8. Sex hormones are used to
   a. replace nutrients in cancer cells.
   b. fight cancer of the prostate and leukemia.
   c. blister the skin.
   d. kill microorganisms.

9. A harmless tumor is
    a. malignant.
    b. cancerous.
    c. benign.
    d. metastasized.
10. The condition known as stomatitis is
    a. inflammation of the stomach membranes.
    b. irritation of the colon.
    c. inflammation of the mucous membranes of the mouth.
    d. none of the above.
11. The discharge of blood or other substances into tissues is
    a. extravasation.
    b. metastasis.
    c. leukopenia.
    d. cytotoxic.
12. Harmful microorganisms are
    a. leukocytes.
    b. cytoplasm.
    c. cells.
    d. pathogens.
13. Proteins that destroy or stop the growth of certain types of microorganisms are
    a. chemotherapy.
    b. antibodies.
    c. leukocytes.
    d. hormones.
14. Seeding cancer cells in other parts of the body is referred to as
    a. benign.
    b. tumor.
    c. metastasis.
    d. harmless.
15. Chemotherapy
    a. is guaranteed to cure cancer.
    b. does not destroy healthy cells.
    c. kills all cancer cells at one time.
    d. can give the patient more years of quality life.
16. Alopecia is
    a. hair loss.
    b. loss of appetite.
    c. extreme fatigue.
    d. tingling of extremities.
17. Vinblastine (*Velban*) and Vincristine (*Oncovin*) are
    a. hormones.
    b. antibiotic antitumor drugs.
    c. miotic inhibitors.
    d. alkylating agents.

18. An immunomodulating agent is
    a. interferon beta-1b.
    b. interferon alpha-2b.
    c. doxorubicin.
    d. interleukin-2.

Match the drug name(s) to the drug family.

______	19. antimetabolites	a. dactinomycin, bleomycin
______	20. alkylating agents	b. fluorouracil, mercaptopurine
______	21. antibiotics used in cancer therapy	c. *Leukeran*, cyclophosphamide, *Mustargen*

When you have passed this mastery test, sign up for a performance test on administering chemotherapeutic agents.

22. White blood cells less than 4000 per mm are
    a. cytostatic.
    b. benign.
    c. metastatic.
    d. leukopenia.
23. You can help your patient receiving an antineoplastic agent by
    a. encouraging the patient to eat red meats.
    b. brushing the patient's teeth with a hard brush.
    c. offering the patient strong smelling foods.
    d. offering the patient a glass of wine with meals.

Name ______________________ Date ______________________ Class ______________

Chapter 19 Test

On the drawing below, name the numbered parts of a needle and syringe.

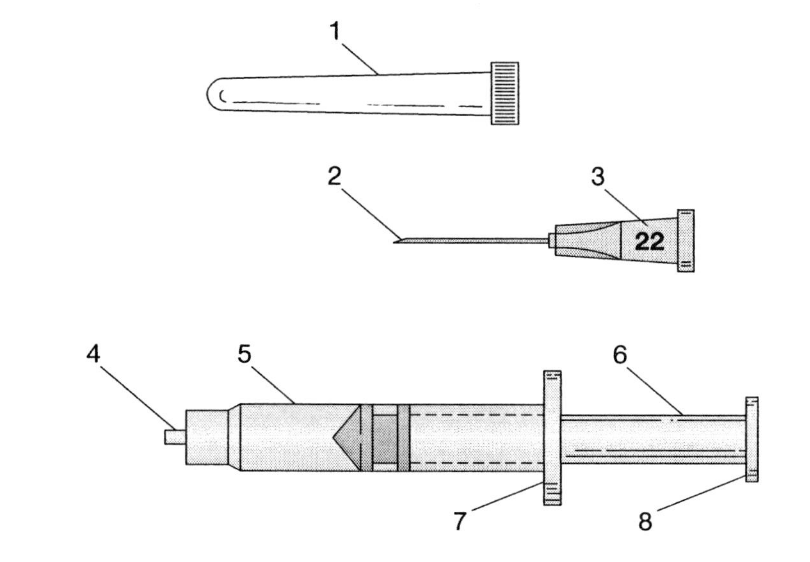

1. ______________________
2. ______________________
3. ______________________
4. ______________________
5. ______________________
6. ______________________
7. ______________________
8. ______________________

Circle the letter of the best choice.

9. Medications may be given parenterally
   a. when a patient has difficulty swallowing or when a patient is vomiting.
   b. when a medication must be absorbed quickly.
   c. when a patient is unconscious.
   d. all of the above.
10. An injection into the fatty layer underlying the epidermis and dermis is referred to as
    a. intradermal.
    b. intramuscular.
    c. subcutaneous.
    d. intravenous.
11. The tapered or slanted portion of an injection needle is called the
    a. hub.
    b. shaft.
    c. flange.
    d. bevel.

12. You are to inject an aqueous medication subcutaneously into an average-sized adult. Which needle is the most appropriate?
    a. 22G $\frac{1}{2}$
    b. 18G2
    c. 26G1$\frac{1}{2}$
    d. 25G $\frac{5}{8}$

13. You have drawn an imaginary line between the greater trochanter and the posterior superior iliac spine. Above and to the outside of this line is the correct location for an injection into the
    a. ventrogluteal site.
    b. dorsogluteal site.
    c. gluteal arteries.
    d. sciatic nerve.

14. The deltoid site differs from other intramuscular sites because it
    a. involves a muscle that may not be well developed in all people.
    b. requires a shorter needle.
    c. is smaller and can absorb less medication.
    d. all of the above.

15. The reason for injecting a measured amount of air into a vial of medications is to
    a. make withdrawing the medications more difficult.
    b. mix the medications with air.
    c. increase the pressure inside the vial.
    d. lessen the pressure inside the vial.

16. On a 3-cc syringe, you count 10 calibration marks between 1 cc and 2 cc. Each mark stands for
    a. 0.1 cc.
    b. 0.2 cc.
    c. 0.5 cc.
    d. 1.0 cc.

17. A new patient is receiving a parenteral medication for the first time. After giving her the injection, you should
    a. leave her alone for an hour so she can get some rest.
    b. stay a few minutes and then stop by frequently to observe for reactions.
    c. stay at her bedside for the next hour.
    d. tell her to press the call button if she feels unusual.

18. You are about to administer an IM injection of an irritating substance. To prevent the tracking of medication into subcutaneous tissue, you may
    a. massage the site vigorously.
    b. have the patient exercise the injected muscle right away.
    c. inject very slowly and wait 10 seconds before withdrawing the needle.
    d. have the patient wear tight-fitting clothing.

19. Adding 0.2 cc of air to a measured dose in a syringe helps to
    a. prevent tracking.
    b. clear the needle of medication.
    c. seal the medication into the tissues.
    d. all of the above.

20. When you perform an intradermal injection properly, you should be able to see
    a. a small blister form just under the skin.
    b. no change in the surface of the skin.
    c. blood in the syringe.
    d. a large lump in the muscle under the skin.

21. You wish to give a patient an intramuscular injection in the vastus lateralis. However, on inspecting the site, you find that the patient's legs are knotted up and sore from a recent football practice. You should
    a. try to inject between the lumpy spots.
    b. select another intramuscular site.
    c. inject the medication intradermally instead.
    d. give the legs a massage and then inject in the vastus lateralis as planned.

22. A patient is ready for the third in a series of injections of an antibiotic. You notice that the spot where you injected her last time is now covered with a fine rash. What should you do?
    a. Do not give the injection, but chart the rash and notify the nurse in charge.
    b. Give the injection in another location that is free of rash.
    c. Give the injection at least one inch away from where the rash ends.
    d. Wait for the rash to clear up and give the injection later.

23. When you aspirate during an intramuscular injection, what does it mean if you see blood in the syringe?
    a. You placed the needle into a blood vessel.
    b. You are properly placed and can proceed with the IM injection.
    c. It is necessary to withdraw the needle slightly and aspirate again.
    d. Both a and c.

24. The proper angle for inserting the needle in subcutaneous injection is
    a. 15°.
    b. 45°.
    c. either 45° or 90°.
    d. 90°.

25. When you place your palm on the greater trochanter and make a "V" with your fingers touching the iliac crest and the anterior superior iliac spine, you have located the
    a. acromion process.
    b. vastus lateralis.
    c. dorsogluteal site.
    d. ventrogluteal site.

26. The "gauge" of a needle is the
    a. hollow part inside the needle.
    b. diameter (width) of the lumen.
    c. length of the shaft.
    d. diameter of the hub.
27. Sloughing, necrosis, and abscess following an injection are signs of
    a. severe tissue damage.
    b. rapid absorption.
    c. improvement in the patient's condition.
    d. systemic reaction.
28. A patient is to be given a medication subcutaneously. It is up to you to select the exact location of the injection. Which are you most likely to choose?
    a. inner lower arm
    b. deltoid muscle
    c. vastus lateralis
    d. upper outer arm
29. When repeated injections must be given, site rotation is practiced because
    a. it allows the dosage to be reduced.
    b. tissue damage can occur with repeated injections in the same place.
    c. the patient may request it.
    d. it helps form scar tissue which makes further injections easier.
30. When giving an injection in the ventrogluteal and dorsogluteal sites, it is important to
    a. avoid hitting the sciatic nerve.
    b. use touch as well as sight to locate the proper site.
    c. place the patient in a position that relaxes the muscles.
    d. all of the above.
31. While injecting *Imferon* by intramuscular route, you use your hand to displace the tissues to one side. You hold the tissues in that position until you withdraw the needle. This is known as the
    a. displacement method.
    b. Z-track method.
    c. tracking method.
    d. site rotation method.
32. You are filling a 100-unit insulin syringe and you wish to measure accurately the ordered dose of 44 units. Between 40 and 50 units you count five calibrations. This tells you that each mark between 40 and 50 measures
    a. 2 cc.
    b. 1 unit.
    c. 2 units.
    d. 0.5 units.
33. A syringe that holds 1.0 cc of medication and is calibrated in hundredths of cc's is a(n)
    a. standard hypodermic syringe.
    b. insulin syringe.
    c. tuberculin syringe.
    d. irrigation syringe.

34. You are concerned about maintaining asepsis so that your patient does not risk infection. In preparing a needle and syringe for injection, you are careful to touch only the
    a. point, hub, outside barrel, and flange.
    b. plunger, shaft, inside needle cover, and plunger.
    c. outside barrel, flange, plunger end, and outside needle cover.
    d. tip, outside needle cover, inside barrel, and hub.
35. Large air bubbles in the syringe
    a. help you measure the dose accurately.
    b. do not affect the injection procedure.
    c. increase the effectiveness of the drug.
    d. should be removed by pointing the syringe straight up and tapping it sharply.

Name ______________________ Date ______________________ Class ______________

Chapter 20 Test

Circle the letter of the best choice.

1. As the body ages,
   a. healing takes longer.
   b. body disorders become less common.
   c. all the systems speed up.
   d. health improves.

2. A patient has a severe case of rheumatoid arthritis and must take several medications every day. His fingers are crippled, but his mind is sharp and he enjoys talking with the nursing home staff about the activities of his college-age grandchildren. There are many tasks, such as dressing and eating, that you must assist him with because of his crippled fingers. You want to help the patient stay as independent and self-confident as possible, so you
   a. take over all the patient's care to save him the trouble.
   b. get the patient to assist you in planning a schedule for his routine medications.
   c. try not to spend much time with the patient because you have so many patients to attend to.
   d. ignore the patient's needs because he is old and will not be around long anyway.

3. When the aging liver and kidneys are slow to metabolize and excrete drugs, there is a danger of
   a. cumulation.
   b. overdose.
   c. toxicity.
   d. all of the above.

4. An eighty-three-year-old patient is new to a long-term care facility. He is to be given a routine dose of liquid aspirin along with several other medications. You know the usual adult dose for aspirin, so you do not check the patient's chart to see what dose has been ordered. In this situation you
   a. showed good judgment because you saved time by not consulting the chart.
   b. showed skill in remembering usual adult doses, so you will rarely need to check patient charts.
   c. showed poor judgment because the aging body demands individualized drug therapy.
   d. saved the patient from possible drug toxicity.

5. Compared to normal adult doses, doses ordered for elderly patients are usually
   a. greater.
   b. smaller.
   c. about the same.
   d. stronger solutions.

6. Which of the following substances, taken together, can lead to drug interactions?
   a. alcohol and sedatives
   b. anticoagulants and phenobarbital
   c. antibiotics and food
   d. all of the above
7. Which of the following statements about aging is true?
   a. It occurs at the same rate in everybody.
   b. The eyes are always the first to go.
   c. The aging body can no longer enjoy sports and sex.
   d. Different parts of the body age at different times in different people.
8. Changes in the gastrointestinal tract of the elderly can lead to
   a. changes in the rate of absorption of nutrients and drugs.
   b. indigestion.
   c. constipation.
   d. all of the above.
9. Drug therapy with the elderly is more complicated than with younger adults because
   a. the elderly are prone to more disorders and therefore take more drugs.
   b. aging bodies are less able to adapt to imbalances caused by drugs.
   c. routine laxatives, antacids, stimulants, and OTC drugs can interact with prescribed drugs.
   d. all of the above.
10. To increase the confidence of your elderly patients,
    a. let them help with administering their own medications if they can.
    b. dress them and feed them yourself because you can do these tasks more efficiently.
    c. whenever possible, avoid talking with them.
    d. treat them as a burden.
11. The study of diseases and disorders in the elderly is called
    a. pediatrics.
    b. podiatry.
    c. geriatrics.
    d. genetics.
12. Eating is often less pleasurable in the elderly because of
    a. inflamed teeth and gums.
    b. loss of the senses of taste and smell.
    c. indigestion caused by changes in the gastrointestinal system.
    d. all of the above.
13. A patient has trouble swallowing pills. To make things easier for the patient, you
    a. crush and mix tablets with applesauce or food as directed.
    b. make sure the patient is lying flat on the back before giving medications.
    c. withhold liquids until the medication is swallowed.
    d. place tablets at the tip of the tongue to promote swallowing.

14. A patient must take several medications at one time, but after the first one or two tablets, the patient refuses to take any more. You should
    a. force the patient to take all the medications.
    b. give the most important medications first.
    c. save the most important medications for last.
    d. skip the patient's medication altogether.
15. A patient has requested a p.r.n. medication, so you check his chart to see if the medication has been given earlier. The chart shows that he has not received a dose of the medication since yesterday. You administer the p.r.n. medication, but in a short while you notice that he was already given a dose of that medication an hour ago. This medication error was caused by
    a. preparing the wrong dose of medication.
    b. inappropriate charting practices.
    c. administering the wrong medication.
    d. the patient's poor judgment.

Place a T in the blank if the statement is true. Place an F in the blank if the statement is false.

______ 16. Flu, pneumonia, and broken bones are more serious for the elderly than for younger persons.

______ 17. The body of an elderly person is better able to handle stress because it has had more experience.

______ 18. Young adults are more likely to have disease complications than the elderly.

______ 19. A decreased supply of oxygen to the brain can be the cause of mental confusion in very old people.

______ 20. Medical staff often find it very rewarding to treat elderly patients because their bodies respond so quickly to medical care.

______ 21. A pill box will organize a patient's pills according to the day to help them remember to take their medicine.

______ 22. The heart and the blood vessels begin to lose their elasticity with aging.

______ 23. Laxatives and anticholinergics affect the absorption of other drugs.

______ 24. You can always safely identify an aged patient by the name on his or her clothes.

______ 25. Timed-released capsules or enteric-coated products should be crushed and mixed with applesauce or similar soft food for an elderly patient who has trouble swallowing or taking medicine properly.